HEALING BREASTFEEDING GRIEF

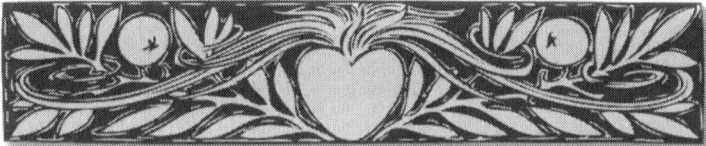

HOW MOTHERS FEEL AND HEAL
WHEN BREASTFEEDING DOES NOT GO AS HOPED

Hilary Jacobson C.Ht

Rosalind Press

Ashland, Oregon

For information, contact motheringinnovations.com

Published by Rosalind Press, Ashland, Oregon

Printed in the United States of America

Library of Congress Cataloging-in-Publication Data

Jacobson, Hilary A.

    Healing Breastfeeding Grief: How mothers feel and heal when breastfeeding does not go as hoped / Hilary Jacobson

Imprint: Mother Food Books Series, Book Two / Rosalind Press

    Summary: "Based on the reported experiences of hundreds of mothers, using processes from neuroscience, somatic therapy, mindfulness and hypnotherapy, and including interviews from mother-baby professionals, practitioners and mothers, *Healing Breastfeeding Grief* speaks to mothers' emotional responses to breastfeeding problems, to the increased risk for postpartum depression and loss of optimal bonding, and shows that breastfeeding grief can be healed when mothers become cognizant of the nature of their grief and receive support, as well as utilizing processes based in neuroscience that allow the brain to heal."—Provided by the publisher

    ISBN: 978-0-9795995-2-1

1. Breastfeeding 2.Postpartum Depression I. Jacobson, Hilary II. Title

First Printing 2016   2016936599

for my mother

Table of Contents

ACKNOWLEDGEMENTS

I would like to thank the mothers who allowed me to support them through their breastfeeding struggles. You showed me how the heart and mind can heal.

I would like to thank the mothers, practitioners and professionals who contributed to this book with interviews and stories. Your knowledge and insights are invaluable.

I would like to thank the mothers from the Yahoo group "MOBI" and the Facebook groups "IGT and Low Milk Supply," "Breastfeeder at Heart," and several non-public Facebook groups (you know who you are) for your heartfelt descriptions of your grieving experiences.

I would also like to thank the writers of the HayWire Writers workshop, Ruth Wire, Joe Suste, Cynthia Rogan, Joshua Hendrickson, and Madeleine Sklar. Your excellent critiques and unabated enthusiasm have been an immeasurable support.

.

INTRODUCTION

If breastfeeding has not gone as planned and hoped, and you are struggling with feelings of loss, sadness, anger, grief or shame, this book is here for you.

These feelings are rarely mentioned in books or childbirth preparation classes. Mothers tend to think they are the only ones feeling this way. But these feelings are not at all unusual. You are not alone.

Fortunately, mothers can heal. This book will assist you on your healing journey.

How to Use This Book

Most of my readers are sleep-deprived and appreciate a little help on how to use this book.

Part One is filled with strategies to guide you toward feeling better.

Part Two leads you through exercises to release anxiety, to relax, and to process your emotions.

Part Three contains interviews with healthcare providers who share their personal and professional experiences with breastfeeding grief.

At the end of Part Three, there are three stories written by mothers who share their struggles with breastfeeding grief, and their healing journeys.

For more information, visit: www.healingbreastfeedinggrief.com

Hilary Jacobson, 2015

Love and Nourishment are One

I still need to hold you near
and feel your dear mouth close
about that tender part of me
where no milk flows.

This sacred thing that should have been,
this rite of every mother,
will not now, nor ever be
a bond, one to the other.

Yet though I feel this utter loss,
a nagging emptiness,
I also smell your warm skin close,
know you don't need me less.

Song and smile, touch and glance,
we dance our dance until –
scent and hand, hold and clasp,
it's clear: I love you still.

If love and nourishment are one,
and I love you just the same,
then let me give you love, my love,
that does not bend to shame.

If love and nourishment are one,
perhaps that's all we need:
to trust our bond is ever here,
regardless how we feed.

-Hilary Jacobson 2004

Part One

First Steps to Healing

THE GIFT OF SELF
NOURISHMENT OF THE HEART

While everyone agrees that breastfeeding is the best way to feed a baby, other kinds of nourishment are also important. How a mother feels, how we are within ourselves as we feed, love, hold and cuddle our baby, is also an essential form of nourishment that only we can give our baby.

During pregnancy, your baby's brain, heart and nervous system are finely attuned to your own.

After birth, your baby's brain, heart, nervous system, immune system, and emotional well-being continue to be attuned to you, and to thrive through the nourishment of your *presence*.

As mothers, we need to ask ourselves if we are *present*—that is, if we are actually *here*, in the moment, mentally and emotionally, with our baby.

The purpose of this book is to help mothers heal from any birth and breastfeeding traumas that prevent us from being present, to help mothers recognize the value of their *very self* for their baby, to help mothers nourish themselves and their baby from their heart.

WHAT IS PRESENCE?

When we were children, we intuitively recognized "presence."

For instance, if we met a grown-up and they leaned in close to say hello, we might have known right away whether we felt comfortable and safe, or if we would rather get away.

Later, in school, we saw how a teacher's presence affected the class. With some, students were naturally cooperative and attentive, but with others, students were chaotic and disrespectful.

I am sure that you can think of many times when you were aware of someone's presence. But what is a person's "presence"?

Philosophers and religious leaders have circled around this question for thousands of years. What is it to be human? To be conscious?

Today's scientists and religious leaders debate these same questions. We're finding out that how we think and feel affects the body, and how we care for and nourish the body affects how we think and feel.

We are discovering that the intestine that digests food also contains tissues and chemicals that are akin to the brain, giving new meaning to the phrase "gut knowing." We know that the heart generates its own electromagnetic field, giving new meaning to "the guidance or voice of the heart." The heart's field, when harmonious, positively affects the brain, hormones and all our internal organs—and it also strengthens our sense of self.

The idea that we have three main centers of "knowing"—brain, heart, and gut—is gaining traction. Mind... feelings... intuitions... As a mother, you will have many opportunities to experience these different parts of your knowing/being over many years to come with your child.

For the purpose of this book, when we speak of "presence," we mean a mother's ability to be comfortable in the here and now. Another way of putting it is that your presence is your ability to settle and relax into the moment and simply *be here*.

Babies *live* in the here and now, and your baby thrives on your presence. Your baby senses your emotions, your nervous system, your anxieties and fears, and also your love, joy, and calm.

Many women say that they do not feel comfortable as a new mother. They might be upset or even traumatized by their pregnancy or childbirth experience. Breastfeeding struggles can be upsetting and traumatizing, too.

Mothers need to find resolution for these feelings so we can relax and be available to our baby and ourselves. Helping mothers resolve these feelings and become confident, comfortable and present is the direction we're headed. So let's get started.

How Did I Get Here?

When breastfeeding challenges arise, the emotions that we feel can be so tumultuous and unexpected that mothers ask: *How did I get here?*

It might have begun like this –

Our initial breastfeeding issues made us concerned.

If we didn't get the answers or support that we needed, we began to feel anxious.

As our problems continued, we may have felt shocked, helpless or afraid, especially if the advice we received was contradictory, or if it did not achieve the hoped-for results.

We may have felt angry—why didn't we know about this ahead of time? Why did no one tell us?

And we may have felt sadness, or shame, or as though we were a failure.

Mothers often say that they are stunned by the intensity of these feelings.

Some say that they don't recognize themself; they are shocked that they could feel this way.

While for some mothers, these feelings lessen with time, for others, they continue and even escalate.

If any of this describes you, please take heart. We are finding ways to heal.

You Can Feel Better

Here are five steps to help you feel better. This is just a summary, an overview of the journey. The next section and the rest of the book contain more detailed information and instructions.

Build your support team

o   Find other women who have gone through similar difficulties. Reach out to friends, family, and professionals. Include your partner in your support team. The section for partners on page 37 is written especially to help your partner appreciate what you are going through.

Understand your issues

o   Find out what caused the problem(s)

o   Understand why it is so emotionally painful

Find remedies if possible for your problems; do what you can to make it right

o   Work with your support team, listen to the wisdom of mothers and the guidance of professionals

o   Be aware of your options and make use of them

Feel and process your emotions

o   Allow tears to flow

o   Find creative expression

o   Dance, walk, move—allow emotions to move through and out of you

o   Do emotional processing (See Part Two)

Focus on the love, on the connected and nourishing relationship that you wish to have with your baby

o   Practice skin-on-skin and heart-to-heart connection

o   Learn infant massage

o   Infant carry, co-sleep or cuddle

o   Practice relaxation exercises and visualizations or mindfulness, and allow these to help you relax and feel close to your baby

HERE ARE YOUR MORE DETAILED INSTRUCTIONS

Find Expert Help. An IBCLC (International Board Certified Lactation Consultant) is your first go-to person. Make an appointment to see the IBCLC who works at your hospital or WIC, look online for local IBCLCs, or get a recommendation for an IBCLC in private practice from your local mothers group.

Look for Peer Support. Join a local and/or online community of breastfeeding mothers. Breastfeeding support groups are found at many hospitals, and there is probably a La Leche League or other peer-support group in your area. Online groups may focus on specific problems, such as mothers who Exclusively Pump, or babies who have Tongue-Tie or GERD-reflux. Finding both a local and an online group is a good way to go. This can relieve feelings of isolation and helplessness.

Organize Your Support Team. Supportive friends and family can help in many ways so you have more time to rest, heal your emotions and mother your baby. Your team will probably also include a breastfeeding expert such as an IBCLC, and any additional practitioners that she recommends. If you have a special relationship to your doula or midwife, stay in contact with them and keep them in your team.

Talk about it. Words of understanding and compassion can go a long way toward helping you feel better. If any people on your team do not understand what you are going through, ask them to read this book, especially the first 40 pages.

If your husband or partner is having a hard time understanding what you are going through, reading or sharing the information in this book may help.

Understand. It is important to understand the reasons behind your breastfeeding challenges. Knowing "why" helps relieve feelings of helplessness.

Write in a journal. Writing frequently about feelings helps us process them. When we sleep at night, our unconscious mind continues processing the emotions and situations that we've written about.

Mothers sometimes find it difficult to journal about their breastfeeding grief. To help you, there is a list of prompts and questions at the end of Part Two.

Express Yourself Creatively. Pent up emotions can flow and be better processed through blogging, photography, drawing, painting, cooking, gardening, writing poetry or stories.

Let your feelings flow into your creative work. If you would like, send me a link to your stories, poetry, photography and artwork. I'd like to see them, and to link to them from my website.

Move your Body. Movement can be soothing, reassuring, and healing. Even surrounded by piles of diapers, mothers can make space to dance a bit, and do some yoga or stretching.

You might also dance while holding your baby, but keep your motions smooth, slow and gentle, and listen to soft music, so that you do not overwhelm your baby's delicate nervous system.

Please remember that you have just gone through pregnancy and birth. Your ligaments need time to pull together, back to their pre-pregnancy tightness and strength. Be careful not to injure yourself by overdoing exercise.

Feel the Baby Love: You might feel judged at times, both by others and by yourself, but please understand that you have given your baby life, and that your baby's heart, brain and nervous system are designed to be in a loving connection with you.

You are surely doing the best for your baby that you can in your situation. Concentrate on this positive sense of yourself as a mother and build that heart-to-heart connection with your baby.

Healing in the Shower. The shower or bath is often the only place where new mothers have a chance of enjoying self-care and pampering. Take advantage of this time. The exercises at the beginning of Part Two will get you started.

THE ORIGIN OF THE TERM "BREASTFEEDING GRIEF"

The phrase Breastfeeding Grief was first used in the early 2000s within the MOBI yahoo-forum.

MOBI stands for Mothers Overcoming Breastfeeding Issues. Our forum was the first online community where mothers could express painful feelings and give and receive support.

While the main issue we saw/see at MOBI is low milk supply, mothers in many different situations share their struggles and their need for emotional healing.

You see, in the early 2000s, breastfeeding experts did not know much about low milk supply, about baby's tongue-tie or about the food allergies and other unusual problems that today are more and more common.

Many professional lactation consultants joined MOBI to lurk in the background and observe how we talked about our problems in a supportive way.

After a few years of pooling our experiences, MOBI moms realized that both mothers and babies were presenting with problems that were not yet recognized in the mainstream.

Many of our babies have tongue- and lip-ties, (Google "tight frenulum and breastfeeding"). Often, when the tie is released, the baby's latch improves and the mother's milk supply increases.

Many of our babies also improve with craniosacral therapy or pediatric chiropracty, which helps babies settle more comfortably into their body.

Mothers with true low milk supply often have hormonal imbalances such as insulin resistance, polycystic ovarian syndrome (PCOS), insufficient glandular tissues (IGT), pre-diabetes, or thyroid issues.

Today, you can read about these subjects on many websites. But it all started through the mothers at MOBI—and this says a lot about the power of online groups to change the way we understand the world.

WISE WORDS OF MOBI MOTHERS

At the MOBI group, mothers often talk about their healing journeys.

In their own voices, here is some of their wisdom:

Breastfeeding after birth is an opportune and unique time for bonding, but it is not the only opportunity or the only way to create deep bonding.

Infant massage and time spent skin on skin and heart-to-heart are other ways.

Bonding is an ongoing process that continues through the life of your relationship. Your emotional healing is ongoing as well.

You are a good and caring mother. Your baby is lucky to have you as their mother.

Reach out to friends and family for support, for instance, ask them to do the shopping or bring you warm meals, so you can relax and have more time for yourself and your baby.

Realize that you need nurturing, care and love. Be gentle with yourself.

Find time to do things that you love, or discover new things to love that you can fit into the time that you have.

At the latest after your child's first birthday, you will feel better. You'll discover a whole new set of activities and pleasures to share with your baby.

It turns out that your baby does not love or need you less, no matter how those initial months went, and this is healing.

BREASTFEEDING AND POSTPARTUM DEPRESSION

In 2014, a British study of 14,000 mothers looked at the effect of breastfeeding grief on the development of postpartum depression (PPD).

They discovered that when mothers who hope to breastfeed are unable to reach their breastfeeding goal, they are *twice* as likely to develop postpartum depression as mothers who succeeded at breastfeeding or mothers who always planned to exclusively use formula,[i]. Even mothers who never experienced depression before were at twice the risk.

This statistic begs the question: How many of these mothers were wrestling with breastfeeding grief? How many could have averted postpartum depression if they had received understanding and support?

From the point of view of mothers at MOBI, one of the main reasons grieving mothers develop postpartum depression is the feeling of being powerless to understand, influence or change their breastfeeding situation.

We have found that when mothers receive a satisfactory diagnosis for their breastfeeding problem and develop a strategy to move forward—they begin to feel optimistic. When mothers change their attitude from *all or nothing* to *willingness to compromise*, say, by topping off their feeds with formula, or feeing with a supplementer at the breast, mothers frequently no longer feel at risk for depression.

It is so important that a mother feels supported as she makes her own best choices, and that she can count on her choices being respected by her spouse, family, friends, healthcare providers, and community of mothers. Unfortunately, mothers often feel that they are blamed or shamed, and not supported. For this reason, online communities that focus on giving respect and support to mothers with breastfeeding challenges are so valuable.

Good nutrition is just as important as information and support. For instance, women in the United States and Canada are often deficient in iron, which leads to fatigue, contributes to depression, and can be a factor for low milk supply. Eating plenty of good, so-called "essential" fats is also helpful, as these fats nourish the brain and nerves, and can make a big difference in how we feel. In my book *Mother Food*, I write about nutritional deficiencies that can affect both a mother's health and her milk supply.

Anyone can suffer from depression. It is a normal reaction to a difficult situation, and does not reflect on a mother personally. If you are feeling at risk for depression, please discuss your situation with your doctor.

Please also understand that depression can sometimes cause mothers to act in ways that they otherwise would not, even harming themselves or their babies. Should you ever have thoughts in this direction, contact your trusted healthcare provider, your midwife, doctor, or therapist, or call 911 or go to your local emergency ward. Don't wait. Get help right away.

HYPNOTHERAPY FOR BIRTH TRAUMA AND BREASTFEEDING GRIEF

While moderating the MOBI group, I listened to hundreds of mothers tell heartbreaking stories.

I often wished for a magic wand that would enable them to move through their trauma and grief so they could enjoy their time with their baby more fully.

My wish was answered when I became certified as a hypnotherapist, and developed a set of inductions to help mothers recover their mothering joy and confidence.

If you would like to try hypnotherapy, contact me through my website, healingbreastfeedinggrief.com.

JOIN A MOTHERS GROUP

It is not unusual for mothers to avoid other mothers. It is a sign of our times. With so many controversial parenting questions in the air, it can be difficult to relax and speak openly except with very good friends.

Controversial subjects include: birth and breastfeeding, circumcision, abortion, schooling, immunizations, television and computer time, the best diet, the best toys, the best everything...

However, these topics fade into the background in a mothers group that is dedicated to breastfeeding problems such as low supply, IGT, D-MER, Tongue-Tie, GERD, Infant Allergies, Healing Breastfeeding Grief and more.

Knowing that others understand and have gone through similar experiences seems to allow mothers to put aside their differences and build a community of support. Giving and receiving can be uplifting. It can be the moment when healing begins.

A Grandmother's Story

A mother told me this story. She is very close to her own mother, and she naturally wanted to tell her about her heartbreaking experience with low milk supply.

As she spoke about it, her mother began to cry.

It turned out that she, too, had struggled with low supply, but had never told anyone about it. Now she could finally grieve.

It is so important that we share our stories and listen to the stories of others. It can mean more than we'll ever know.

In Mothers' Own Words

I asked mothers in online groups to describe the emotions of breastfeeding grief. Their accounts may be shocking to some readers. Yet, knowing how other mothers feel can be helpful. You can truly know you are not alone.

Some of these mothers, just starting out, are emotionally bleeding and raw. Others, looking back, are able to express appreciation for what they have learned and gained throughout their healing journey.

If reading these quotes is uncomfortable, feel free to skip this section. Another option: I have put the mothers' positive thoughts in italics. If you wish, you can skim through and read these bits exclusively.

Christina

I sobbed for hours! Nothing could take away the feelings of guilt, worry and rejection. It affected my relationship with my new baby. I was so preoccupied and I missed so much in those early days! I felt isolated and alone.

Things are better now. There is hope! And I know my baby loves me even though breastfeeding has been a struggle, one of the greatest of my life.

Arielle

I could only produce 50% of my baby's needs. Dark thoughts and negative self-talk made me feel that I had failed my son, that I was unfit to mother. Not only did obesity cripple my self-esteem, but those first three exhausting months completely undermined my self-worth.

I tracked every single drop of his intake and output on charts for 10 months out of hypervigilence. Then I started to understand and research, look for and find support.

This journey has changed me to my core. Now I love myself, I love my body. I'm taking what I've learned about why I experienced suppressed lactation and using that knowledge to heal my body. This journey has been a lifesaver and I would not have it another way.

I feel so much empathy for women in the early throes of it, it's emotionally crippling and combined with those postpartum hormones and sleep deprivation, it's akin to surviving emotional warfare with ourselves. I am eternally grateful for this online community's help through an emotional nursing journey and now a wonderful weight loss journey.

Nicole

I felt so much self-hatred. I once punched myself repeatedly in my breasts. I was disgusted with their inability to feed my failure-to-thrive child or to letdown to the pump. I was sick of having unexplainable plugged ducts and mastitis. My breasts were my enemy. This was before I knew that a posterior tongue-tie was causing every one of these issues.

To this day I get sick with guilt thinking of the hypoallergenic formula I was forced to give my failure-to-thrive baby for nine months while I worked through major breastfeeding issues. He was so unbelievably sick and became sicker every day. This was because he had an unknown corn allergy; the first ingredient in his formula.

Elizabeth

I felt such a great weight of sadness in the early days that I was completely buried in it. *I still feel sadness for that time, but more as compassion now.*

I went through a process of grief and mourning that changed subtly over time throughout the first year of our breastfeeding journey. I blamed and hated myself in the first few months to a degree that I found shocking, even in the midst of it. We went through a lot to get pregnant, and I remember in that first month, struggling to feed her, having persistent thoughts about how I shouldn't have been a mother.

Anxiety plagued me like crazy in the first months. I worried about all the things I probably should have done differently, I worried about the scads of pro-breastfeeding articles I'd read while I was pregnant. And I worried every time I needed to nurse in public that people were secretly judging me.

To end on something positive, though, I feel amazing to have persevered through that first year.

I'm a social worker, but if time and money allowed I would love to go back to school to get certified as an IBCLC, postpartum doula, baby-wearing instructor...I could have a whole different career.

Salwa

I feel jealous that others can breastfeed so easily and boast about it while us less fortunate mothers struggle and put ourselves through so much heartache and stress. I sometimes look at my daughter and resent her for not wanting my breast although there is milk there. I resent her for not suckling properly, and I then resent myself for feeling that way towards her, and not being able to provide for her the way I so desperately want to.

Lea

I work at a breastfeeding support center. To help moms thrive while I couldn't help myself was an emotional roller coaster. In the beginning I was angry. I didn't find it fair that I spent my first few weeks literally in bed skin-to-skin with my newborn and he still wasn't gaining. I was jealous that other moms could leave the house while for me, nursing, then pumping, then hand expressing around the clock consumed all of my thoughts and actions. After the anger passed, I just felt heartbroken.

It took a donor mom's help to heal my heart.

Beth

In those early weeks I felt my grief in my chest like a hollowness, an ache. The hopefulness that is a new baby, combined with the emptiness of my breasts, the fullness of my heart, and the "overwhelmyness" of my brain/hormones was something I'll never forget.

Rosie

For a long time I felt angry at my body and God that I had been cheated of the opportunity to exclusively breastfeed my son.

Over time I became brazenly open about my low supply and unapologetic. I found peace with it and made it my mission to support other low supply mamas and help them feel less alone and ashamed.

Laura

When breastfeeding my first son, if he latched painfully I wouldn't take him off and re-latch. I would tell myself I deserved the pain and then make myself endure my 'punishment' for not making enough milk for him. It was a very dark place for me.

Lisa

Sometimes I'd just stand in the mirror staring at my breasts trying to understand how they could fail both myself and my son this way. I had learned that I had breastfeeding failure and was supplementing donor milk with an SNS. I was crushed and felt like a complete failure of a woman. It took weeks to not cry about it at the drop of a hat.

Sami

I labeled myself a failure and even thought, "I'm not a REAL mother," which I now know is absurd. I struggled immensely with feeling envious of women who could breastfeed. Envy is so much more toxic than jealously to me. Jealously is wishing that I can have what you have. Envy has an element of wanting to take away or spoil what the other person has and thinking that I deserve it more than they do.

So for me, I couldn't be happy for my friends who were nursing their babies. This is not who I am at all, so then I'd feel guilty on top of everything else. It was a vicious cycle of guilt and shame.

Rachel

I typically feel broken and exhausted. I feel consumed by the need to try and force something I may not be able to control no matter what. It makes you desperate. The exhaustion comes from all the hours of extra feedings, pumping, and then feeding formula if necessary. You never sleep and when you have a break, it's booked with appointments or reading or trying to get more help. And you're always under the gun because the clock is always ticking on the next meal, the next reminder that no matter how much you want to give this sweet little person the best start and fulfill a basic human need, that you're just broken. Other people make you feel stupid or lazy, like you haven't tried EVERYTHING already...or you're not trying hard enough. You begin to not feel human from the lack of sleep and trying so hard...and then you're too overwhelmed to enjoy this beautiful miracle. This was not how I imagined my start to motherhood.

Richanna

Guilt. I suffered with large breasts my whole life. Back problems and being "the girl with big boobs" were the reasons at the top of my list to get breast reduction at age 20. The doctor told me I would be able to breastfeed if I ever had children. Technically, I guess he was right. I CAN breastfeed; but following it with a bottle of formula was not what I had in mind. I got the surgery and have never regretted it until the birth of my son. For months, I felt guilty because I felt I put my health concerns before his, even though he wasn't here at the time of my decision.

But I exclusively-pumped for 6 months, and with the help of support sites was producing 75% of my baby's needs! So after the fact... I feel PROUD. I stuck with it (even if just for 6 months) and gave my baby 100% of what I could, when I could have much easier given up!

Hilary's request for comments allowed me to begin expressing my feelings, and that was part of the healing process in coming to terms with my struggling breastfeeding journey.

Brittnae

I would let myself have a few moments of mourning each day while I was in the shower. I would sit and sob and let the water wash it all down the drain... then I would pick myself up and go love my baby like I was meant to. My breasts didn't work, but my mother's heart did.

Holly

I remember thinking, "Maybe I should try harder. Maybe I'm not doing xyz right. Maybe the next feeding will work." And then I'd hook up to my pump because I was scared, scared to hear her cry while trying to latch, scared that it wouldn't work and I'd be reduced to tears again for the hundredth time. Eventually, I gained a new mantra. *"What is the most important thing? That she EATS. Does it matter HOW she eats? No. Does it matter WHAT she eats? No. Just. That. She. Eats."*

Melinda

Frustration. I remember feeling so frustrated with my little tiny baby that JUST WOULD NOT GO TO SLEEP! She would just cry in my arms for hours. I actually felt as if I was losing my mind. I remember that, after hours of trying one day in particular, I left her in the middle of my bed and went into my ensuite, screamed as loud as I could into a towel, and then banged my head into the wall and hit the wall repeatedly. Looking back that sort of behavior out of frustration also caused/causes me to feel guilt, shame, self-blame, self-hatred, regret and sadness.

Marina

I think the shame and the self-blame have been the hardest for me. I was so determined to exclusively breastfeed my twins and I felt like my body failed and let down my whole family. It somehow felt like something I should have been able to control or make my body do, and that I just wasn't strong enough or determined enough to force my body into producing more.

When other mothers talk about feeling sorry for babies who are fed formula it feels like a physical blow. I felt too ashamed to attend breastfeeding support meetings and I hated people asking if I breastfed because I felt like a fraud. Like I wasn't a real breastfeeding mother. I felt so ashamed of my body's failure to feed my children.

WHY WE GRIEVE SO MUCH

Some mothers, reading this book, will say, "Really? Do we really need an explanation? Isn't it completely obvious?"

They might say, "I just carried my baby within my body for nine months! I watched my belly grow and I gave birth! I was all set to breastfeed my baby—to provide all of my baby's nourishment from my own body. Now I am beyond heartbroken."

But while for some, the reasons are obvious, for others, the heartbreak is perplexing. It seems out of proportion to the actual events, somehow.

They might ask, "Aren't we making too much of this? Being childish? Ungrateful?"

Explanations such as "hormones and sleep-deprivation" provide some comfort, but they also leave us unsatisfied.

Surely there is more to it.

In the next three sections you can read some theories as to why we possibly feel as badly as we do. Perhaps you will find some answers for your own situation in these sections, or be inspired to find your own interpretation.

ONE THEORY: THE INSTINCT TO MOURN

In 2009, a group of researching psychologists asked this question: Why do women grieve so much when their breastfeeding hopes and plans are disappointed[ii]?

Here is the answer they found: When a mother is unable to breastfeed, it is possible that her brain, which is imprinted with ancient and primal patterns, actually believes that she has lost her baby.

The researchers explain that for thousands of years, if a woman did not nurse her baby, it was probably because her baby had not survived.

They theorize that when we do not succeed at breastfeeding, a very old part of the brain believes we are in mourning.

Some mothers do describe their breastfeeding grief as akin to having lost a loved one. With the rational part of their brain they know that their baby is alive and well. But emotionally, they struggle with a sense of bereavement that feels absolutely real.

ANOTHER THEORY: A MOTHER'S BRAIN SOUNDS THE ALARM

To understand this next theory, let's first take a step back and look at how the brain works.

As humans, the outer layer of our brain (cerebral cortex) is highly developed. This thinking part of the brain enables us to be problem solving and to use language. However, this is only a small part of the brain, a small part of who we are.

Older parts of the brain are instinctual. Their job is to ensure our survival and they do that by marking dangerous situations with stark emotions, such as pain or fear. For instance, you only need to touch a hot stove once, and a memory of the pain prevents you from doing it again.

The instinctual brain is always on the alert for danger. This is why, even if we love flowers, if we see flowers and a tiger in the same meadow, our brain tells us to run away.

Instinctive reactions are so important that they may even be imprinted in our DNA. Spiders and snakes can be deadly, and some people are born with a profound fear of these creatures. They inherit this fear as a *genetic memory*.

Could it be that strong emotional reactions to breastfeeding problems are a genetic memory as well? Could they be part of our mothering instinct?

Of course they are! These emotions alert the mother to danger, and ensure the survival of her baby.

If a baby is unhappy at the breast (crying too much, drinking too little, unable to latch or suckle well), a mother's brain will respond by firing off anxiety and confusion. These emotions are a signal of *red alert*; they push a mother to respond to her child's distress, to figure out what is going on.

In earlier societies, mothers would immediately turn to other mothers for advice and support. Another woman might even breastfeed her baby until her problems were solved.

In today's society, we don't have a tribe of mothers close by who can give us advice or share breastfeeding duties. Just the opposite: days might pass before we find the advice and support we need. During this time, the brain continues to sound the alarm, and it might even turn up the volume.

To the mother, unable to quickly fine the support, understanding and direction that she needs, it can feel as though her brain is stuck in emergency mode. As her panic and helplessness escalate, she may become worn down and exhausted by her emotions. This puts her at risk for chronic anxiety and/or postpartum depression.

It is good to know that practices of focused relaxation and mindfulness are remarkably successful at turning off the brain's alarm system and restoring peace and quiet to the mind and heart. You can learn more about this in Part Two.

AT THE HEART OF OUR GRIEF

The first three months after childbirth are a magical and challenging time. So much is new! Babies enter the world and they breathe, cry, drink, digest, urinate and defecate for the first time on their own. Babies also learn how to relax and feel safe in their mother's arms, and how to sleep for the first time on a solid surface. Life is filled with new smells, illuminated by electric lights and computer screens, and is loud with ringtones of phones, the sounds of traffic, and the abrupt and confusing sounds of entertainment.

But babies are not the only ones who are adapting to a new situation. As mothers, we also go through a transitional time. Our body heals. We shed extra fluid, our connective tissues start tightening up again, and our hormones first overwhelm us and then begin to even out.

As well as these physical changes, we undergo powerful emotional changes. For many months, we shared our physical space, our air, nutrition, brain chemistry and hormones with our baby. The loss of the indescribable oneness of pregnancy—even though it was not always comfortable—takes getting used to.

With my first baby, I was too overwhelmed with the excitement and newness of motherhood to understand how much I was hurting in this regard. But with my later children, I felt it keenly. The intimate and incomparable presence of my baby within my body was missing. Sometimes, I thought that if I concentrated, I could still feel traces of my baby inside me, as if he had left something behind—a handkerchief maybe, or an old love-letter. That is what it felt like: my beloved had moved out but left little bits to remember him by.

Today, we know that traces of the unique DNA of each of our children do in fact continue to live on within us, to become part of our body. I still remember the day I first read about that. Even though years had passed, it made me happy to know that their DNA continued to be inside me.

I cannot remember reading anything in breastfeeding books about how breastfeeding helps a mother heal from separation after childbirth.

Yet it is obvious: When we breastfeed, we hold our baby close for hours and hours each day. We are connected by the physical flow of milk, and by the hormonal changes that support an emotional flow of tenderness. Clearly, this intense physical contact between a baby and mother is important to a mother's well-being, and it should come as no surprise that mothers with breastfeeding challenges say, simply: "I am heartbroken."

Breastfeeding is supposed to be our path into motherhood. Now what do we do?

In all of history, there is no story that tells mothers what to do, emotionally, mentally or spiritually, when their most biologically natural path into motherhood is jeopardized or lost.

But while lack of "story" is part of our struggle, it is also an opportunity: we can create a new "hero's journey." By applying what we know today about healing from trauma and grief, we can forge a path from the heart of our grief to the heart of our joy—because we *can indeed heal* when we realize that it is our loving presence, most of all, which nourishes a baby and allows a mother's brain and heart to heal.

Just holding your baby and coming into the present moment close allows love to flow between you. This is what you want to salvage—this essential bond, your unique connection.

Regardless of how a mother feeds her baby, when we cultivate heart to heart connection and experience the value *of our very self* for our baby, we can recover our confidence and travel our path into motherhood—with a new and wonderful feeling of wholeness and self-worth.

What You Can Do

Use every opportunity to experience closeness with your baby.

Try co-sleeping (read how to do it safely).

Try co-bathing (read how to do it safely).

Sign up for a course in infant massage, which has many of the benefits of breastfeeding. In Part Three, read about infant massage with JoAnn Lewis.

Cuddle together beneath a blanket. (Be certain that your baby has an open flow of air and can breathe freely.)

Even if there is little or no milk flowing, if your baby will accept your breast, "breast-nurturing" can be a source of comfort.

If you bottle feed, create a quiet place where you feel safe and comfortable, and hold your baby close to your body, just as you would when breastfeeding. Keep eye contact with your baby, and allow yourself to feel the flow of connection.

The visualizations in Part Two, especially *Wrap Your Baby with Love*, will help build this connection.

ADVICE FOR YOUR PARTNER

When we find ourselves in a situation that is much more difficult than we expected it to be, it is tempting to want to simplify things, to remove the complicating factors, in this case, to say, "If breastfeeding isn't easy, stop trying."

This is the "helpful advice" that many spouses offer their wives when the attempt to breastfeed is obviously a struggle. They don't want to see their wife feel bad, and they themselves are pained by her struggle.

However, there is no guarantee that stopping will improve the situation. It could make it worse—and it often does.

Your partner must find her own best path into motherhood. Even with added difficulties, learning about options and making her own best choices is important to her long-term healing.

What you can do: support her with your words and with actions. If you have time, help around the house, prepare healthy snacks and beverages, and shop and prepare meals—or contact friends and family to help out.

When you share time with your spouse and your baby, try not to expect her to be any different than she is, or that she feel better than she does. Appreciate your new life just as it is, messy house, emotional wife and all.

Your transition into parenthood is important. You are important to your wife and your child in ways that may be new to you. There are online groups and books and podcasts that talk about your transition. Find other parents and talk through your joys and challenges. Be good to yourself.

Trauma and the Brain

According to two studies, about a third of mothers report having symptoms of posttraumatic stress disorder (PTSD) after giving birth, though only about 3% have it severely[iii].

As we now know, breastfeeding challenges can be traumatizing as well.

But what does that mean, to have symptoms of trauma?

When we are traumatized, we aren't able to put the experience behind us. A part of us seems stuck in the event that caused the pain, *as if it were happening now.*

For mothers, this means that trauma interferes with our ability to be present and emotionally accessible both to our baby and to ourself. A part of us is frozen.

The brain actually changes when we endure trauma. Certain parts of the brain become more active, and others, less active. We become less flexible, less able to take in new information.

Sometimes, new trauma builds upon older trauma. It's possible that the initial trauma happened so long ago that we no longer remember what caused it. Yet, it predisposes us to be more sensitive to new trauma in our present life.

Scientists also talk about "generational trauma," that is, about the impact that the experiences of past generations have on future generations.

Clearly, we need to take mothers' traumas seriously. We need to do everything we can to both prevent trauma and to respond to it as quickly as possible so that it can resolve and heal.

I feel immense gratitude that mothers today can learn deep relaxation, mindfulness, and similar processes that actually help the brain heal from trauma.

I advocate that mothers receive such training as a preventative before and during pregnancy, and again, after birth.

In Part Three, Chanti Joy Smith talks about her work with birth trauma, and Anna Humphreys shares how mothers report very little childbirth trauma—even with a difficult or emergency childbirth—when they practice *Calm Birth* meditation during pregnancy.

COMPLEXITIES OF BREASTFEEDING GRIEF

When grief is entangled with emotions such as guilt, anger, blame, shame and remorse, the grief is more challenging to move through. The medical term for this is *complicated grief* or *complex grief.*

Breastfeeding grief is a clear example of complicated grief, and untangling and resolving our emotions can be a challenge.

It helps to think of these emotions as a response to complex pressures, both internal and societal.

We have already talked about internal pressures: about basic survival instincts, about the need of a mother's heart to nourish her baby, and about how breastfeeding offers a biologically natural transition from the oneness of pregnancy into the twoness of motherhood.

External societal pressure is different. It harks from everything we have read or heard over the span of our lifetime that makes us feel that are not a good or true mother if we do not breastfeed.

Tragically, society's voices become internalized, that is, we come to fully believe and identify with their messages. Now, if breastfeeding doesn't work out, a part of us might actually believe that we are the worst possible mother, and that we deserve to feel bad.

Society's voices can lose their power over us when we comprehend that the essence of nurturing and bonding takes place through our loving presence and our touch, regardless how we feed.

Consider this: mothers who succeed at breastfeeding might still be emotionally distant and unavailable to their baby. A perfect breastfeeding relationship does not guarantee perfect bonding, and these mothers, too, may need help overcoming whatever is in the way of their being comfortable and present in the here and now with their baby.

Your baby needs you to be an anchor to his or her growing sense of self. You become an anchor through your presence, your loving touch, and through heart to heart connection. Breast milk cannot replace that essential sustenance. There is no substitute for your heart.

Please, do not mistake breastfeeding success with success as a mother.

My Personal Experience with Breastfeeding Grief

I should have had a good milk supply. My doctor and lactation expert agreed that I was doing everything right, that my baby's latch and suck were correct, strong and effective.

But if that were true, why was my baby so unhappy at the breast?

It turns out that I had a moderate case of insufficient mammary tissue and that my hormones were out of balance.

At that time, very little was known about these issues and their influence on milk supply.

Here is what happened.

As the days and weeks passed, it was obvious to me that nursing was not going well. After the initial letdown, my always-hungry son would pull and tug at my breast, as if working hard for every drop. Then he'd wrench his head away from my breast and scream in complete frustration.

When I turned to them for help, both my lactation expert and pediatrician asked if I fed on demand. When my answer was yes, they assured me that I must therefore have a sufficient supply.

As I continued to struggle to breastfeed my baby, I prayed each day that my efforts would finally yield the desired result, that I would wake up tomorrow and breastfeeding would be as it should be. But each day the frustration continued, and I sank deep into breastfeeding grief.

I had hoped that breastfeeding would be joyful. I knew that the hormones of milk production help mothers be calm and feel joy, and I wanted to feel that.

I hoped breastfeeding would be a time of trust. I wanted to trust my body to provide nourishment for my baby.

I hoped breastfeeding would build my self-confidence and ensure our bonding. My relationship to my own mother hadn't been the best; I was counting on breastfeeding to show me and my baby a way to experience the closeness that I hadn't had with my own mother.

Indeed, some mothers do say that breastfeeding brings them this kind of emotional healing. As they bring their love to their baby, they feel as though they can bring love to their own inner infant-self, and soothe feelings of neglect, abandonment or abuse. I have to admit, I hoped for that kind of healing.

Unfortunately, breastfeeding did not give me joy, calm, healing or self-confidence. As my hope turned to sorrow, I was convinced of my failure as a mother.

My son was four months old and no longer gaining weight when I bought a package of formula and prepared his first bottle. His face lit up with satisfaction as he drank, and I was devastated. Not only had I failed at breastfeeding, but by trying so hard to exclusively nurse I had missed out on a less frustrating and doubtless more bonding experience.

At that time, no one spoke about low supply. There were no support groups, no explanations, and no help. I felt isolated, abandoned, and hopeless.

My healing began while breastfeeding my second son. That is when I realized with amazement that what I ate and drank had an influence on my ability to produce enough milk, and also to produce milk that was easy for my baby to digest.

It turns out that women around the world know about these foods and herbs, but in the West, this knowledge has not been studied. I decided to do my best to make this information available to others. When I *re-purposed* my grief into a goal to help others, I began to derive a sense of purpose and meaning from my painful experience. I was on the road to feeling better.

TODAY, MANY OPTIONS FOR SUPPORT

Today, mothers have options that just a decade or two ago did not exist. If you think about it, each of these options is the result of a mother's grief, healing, and re-purposing of her experience in the service of others.

Here are a few examples.

o You have childbirth choices.

o You can hire a birth and/or postpartum doula.

o You can take relaxation trainings such as yoga, Calm Birth Meditation, and Hypnobirthing.

o You can create a detailed postpartum plan

o You can have your support team already in place.

o You can receive physical therapy that enables you and your baby to heal the physical traumas of birth.

o You can work with practitioners who specialize in emotional trauma.

o You can join a mothers group online and receive support and information.

o You can use a supplementer at the breast while building your supply.

o You can look for a milk donor.

o You can choose formulas that are homemade or that use quality ingredients.

And yet, even with all these options, many mothers still feel alone and without support in the weeks following childbirth.

The problem seems to be that when we are pregnant, we are unable to realize just how much in need of assistance and support we will be. It is often not until we are sleep-deprived and emotionally fried that we recognize what we need.

If this describes you, please know that you have options that can make a difference to your life now.

Join a mothers group and ask for information. The more you find out about your options, the more sense of control, competence and community support you can have, and this goes a long ways toward feeling better.

STARTING TO HEAL

Mothers often say they regret not being able to enjoy this precious time with their newborn more fully, and they wish they could do the first weeks over again.

While it is true that we cannot go back, we can decide to move forward into a better state of mind now, as smoothly and quickly as possible.

For this, though, we first need to allow ourselves to feel what we feel.

This may sound odd, but only by allowing our emotions to come to the surface and expressing our emotions through movement, by putting them into a journal, talking about them with someone who understands, or letting our tears flow, can we begin to feel better.

More about this in the next section.

ALLOW YOUR EMOTIONS

Many people are not very skilled when it comes to dealing with painful emotions. We don't really learn this at school! Because feelings can seem so overwhelming, we resist feeling them. But the energy we use to resist and to push our feelings down actually makes them feel even more overwhelming. To understand this, imagine pushing a beach ball under water: the harder you push it down, the more force it seems to exert back to the surface. That is how it can be with emotions, too. Only if we stop pushing them down can they surge up to the surface, and we can feel them fully.

Another way to think about emotions is to imagine them as waves rolling onto a beach. Seen from a distance, waves appear large and powerful. But as they roll on to the shore, they are just a gentle flow. In the same way, if we keep our emotions at a distance, they can seem huge and overwhelming. But by intentionally allowing them in, they become more manageable.

Now, when emotions are held back for a long time, they don't just go away. They simmer beneath the surface and often make themselves a home in the body. For instance, we might feel them as a lump in the throat, as a constriction of the chest, as a pain in the heart area, and as knots in our shoulders. They might express themselves as lower back pain, as headaches or digestive issues such as IBS. Remarkably, each of these health conditions responds very well to hypnotherapy. Through guided trance, we can identify, process and resolve the original emotions.

If you are struggling to feel and be present with your emotions, I suggest that you start with the Focused Relaxation exercises in Part Two.

REFRAME YOUR STORY

Reframing is an effective and straightforward process that is often used in therapy. You can do it on your own, too.

To reframe means to re-tell an old story with a new and positive meaning, interpretation, or outcome. The key to a good reframe is that the new story should feel right; it should ring true to you.

You should be able to believe your reframe.

Guiding your brain to discover a new and positive interpretation is a good first step toward feeling better. When we sincerely look for a positive meaning to life's events, our brain and body respond with positive ideas and feelings.

You may have heard about gratitude journaling, which is a kind of reframing. By recording something we are grateful for every day, our mind becomes sensitized toward that which we value in life, toward that which brings us happiness.

It doesn't matter at all whether the thing we are grateful for is large or small, or if it is material, emotional, or spiritual. Simply viewing our life with gratitude moves us into a positive state of mind. It makes us receptive to positive changes, and we discover that we have more to be grateful for.

When you reframe your breastfeeding story, you will want to think about your reframe-story many times a day. Try writing your reframe-story on a card and placing it where you nurse. Read your new story frequently; take pleasure in it; let it run through your mind and evoke pleasant images.

Reframing Examples:

o   Being sad makes me feel honest deep down inside myself. It may sound strange, but I actually see more clearly how much I care about my baby through how sad I've been. I want to use every moment to be a loving mother to my baby. I love my baby so much.

o   I am learning visualizations for heart-to-heart-connection, and I notice how this is helping me feel better, more connected with my baby and also with other family members. It is good to see something positive come of this.

o   While I wouldn't wish it on anyone, you really can go through breastfeeding grief and come out on the other side as a more mature and understanding person, more sympathetic toward the suffering of other people. I used to be much more judgmental, and now I just want to understand and be kind.

o   All my life, I've been guilting myself, asking, *Why me?* and coming up with lots of self-blaming explanations. I guilted myself for this, too, but then I realized that my baby needs me to be positive. I've been practicing self-forgiveness and feel much better about myself.

o   I have been suffering with D-MER, and learning breathing techniques has helped me deal with the difficult physical and emotional feelings. While I wouldn't want anyone to go through this, I was able to take some important lessons from it. I'm seeing how being in the moment and focusing on my breath allows me to be less affected by passing feelings.

Remember: The new, positive meaning must ring true to you. By telling and retelling your new stories, you generate the positive feelings they evoke. After some time, you might share your new, positive story with friends and family, and with a trusted community of mothers.

This is your healing story.

Your Positive Future Focus

A common experience of early motherhood is nostalgia for the past. We yearn to get back to "who I used to be," to have our former body back again, to have a full night's sleep, to enjoy uninterrupted time with our partner. We yearn to reclaim our "old life."

It is true that it takes time to be comfortable in our new life as a mother. It is also true that time seems to pass so slowly during the initial weeks with a baby, and that the weight of that time, spent repetitiously in feeding and caring for a baby, can be daunting. (In hindsight, of course, it will all seem to have gone by unspeakably fast.)

But although we cannot go back to who we were before we were pregnant, we can turn our focus toward the future, toward the person we are becoming, the mother we are becoming.

Such "future focus" is an important part of therapy. By looking forward to who we are becoming, we have more energy and zest for the present moment. We have more patience, are more creative, and more willing to meet our challenges.

Looking forward to who we are becoming, we can treasure and explore this time with our baby.

o   For instance, you can make a baby diary and look forward to the time when these notes and photos will be precious memories.

o   You can sort through your clothing and give yourself permission to be who you are now, without judgment, while also looking forward to your body in the future.

o   You can join mothers' groups locally and online, and look forward to making friends who understand the new you.

o   You can learn ways to reduce your baby's colic or stomach upset, and you can look into healthy food and meals that you plan to serve your baby when he or she is older.

o   If you have not already done so, you can read through websites or books on immunizations. You can look forward to making informed choices for your family.

o   As you are doing all this, you can be healing your emotions and you can look forward to feeling better and better.

Touch: Our Key to Connection

I recently read a funny valentine card online: "You are my favorite person to lie next to in bed while we look at our phones."

In today's world, many of us are accustomed to a life with little touch. However, as a mother (and of course also as a father), it is essential to literally "be in touch" with your baby. Touch is, after all, your baby's first language. It is the way your baby feels connected to the world.

Physical connection through touch allows two nervous systems to line up and be aware of each other. For instance, a tender hug can allow two persons to sense each other deeply. This may sometimes be so tangible that it seems as though we feel the bio-energy flowing through one another's bodies.

Your touch is your baby's primary nourishment. A study of babies in orphanages in wartime showed that even if babies received enough food, if they did not feel a bond to another person through being touched and held, they died.

One study on babies in NICU showed that the gentle touch of the mother's fingers on the baby, not stroking or massaging, just the mere touch, enabled those babies to gain weight twice as quickly as babies who did not receive touch.

Your touch enables your baby to feel whole. It says, "You are welcome in this world. You are not alone, and you are safe. You can expand and grow. I am here for you."

Skin-to-Skin

You've heard about skin-to-skin contact, about how your baby's naked skin against your own triggers a cascade of hormones and neurochemicals for bonding and connecting—for both of you.

Please practice skin-on-skin every day with your baby, as often and long as possible.

Remove your top and bra, undress your baby, (perhaps leaving the diaper on, or a diaper or towel close by), and hold your baby on your chest while sitting up or lying down.

If the air is at all chilly, cover your baby with a blanket. Always leave your baby's nose uncovered and free to breathe.

You might also want to have a "baby moon" in which you stay in bed all day with your baby, allowing yourself to be served and supported by family and friends, as you give yourself and your baby this special time together.

As you lay together, skin on skin, you might want to practice one of the focused-relaxation, mindfulness or visualizations that you can read about in Part Two. Soon you'll be able to easily forget about the time and sink into the "zone" of gentle connection with your baby.

HEART-TO-HEART

Babies hunger for the flow of emotional warmth that emanates from their parent's hearts. And this is not mere poetry. Researchers have discovered that as the heart pumps blood, it generates an actual electro-magnetic field that is measurable. If you feel relaxed and safe, positive and well, your heart's energy field becomes smooth and harmonious. This is called a coherent field.

Because the heart's field is the most powerful in the body, your brain's energy field will line up with your heart—not the reverse. This is why people say we should "follow our heart" and that the "heart's voice is true."

The heart is the point of authenticity within us. It is also the fulcrum of meditation, prayer and self-healing.

While these few paragraphs only provide a short overview of what is known today about the heart's energy field, it is enough to help us appreciate what this can mean to us as parents.

Simply holding your baby on your chest skin-to-skin, and enjoying shared time together can connect you heart-to-heart with your baby.

The more you come into the present moment, allowing your breath to slow down and deepen, not thinking, not worrying, but being present in the here and now, the more the energy field of your heart becomes coherent, that is, smooth and harmonious. As your baby's energy field lines up with your heart's energy field, you'll feel how your baby relaxes and settles.

It is this coherent alignment, heart-to-heart, that gives your baby feelings of safety and connectedness.

You can be proud and happy to know that when you give your baby the essential "comfort food" of your heart, you support your baby's physical and emotional health, you strengthen your baby's immune system, and you give yourself and your baby an experience that helps bond you more securely together.

TRIGGERS, DIFFICULT EMOTIONS AND SITUATIONS

Even when mothers feel better, certain situations can trigger the return of negative feelings. This will doubtless happen to you at one time or another. When it does, having read about it first here will help you move through the emotions more quickly.

o   For instance, you might feel upset when you see other mothers breastfeed, apparently without issue.

o   You might feel upset when bottle feeding or using an SNS in public if you receive stares, remarks or questions as to why you are not breastfeeding.

o   You might feel upset if you meet mothers who could easily breastfeed but choose not to.

o   There will also be triggers that are specific to your situation.

o   For instance, if your baby was failure-to-thrive, seeing a photo of that time can bring up bad feelings, or seeing other babies who are clearly thriving can bring up the sadness and grief.

To find relief when you are triggered, connect with mothers who have walked in your shoes. Hearing, "I know what you are feeling, I've been there, too," is soothing. You are not alone.

In the following sections, we will look at potential triggers in detail.

CONCERN ABOUT FORMULA

For mothers who need to supplement with formula, brand name formulas are often the most available and affordable choice. Yet, for mothers who hoped to exclusively breastfeed, the necessity of having to use these products can evoke very negative feelings.

The solution here is to rethink and soften our attitude, in other words, to do a reframe exercise around formula.

For instance, we can appreciate and be grateful for all the good science and regulation that has gone into making formula as healthful and safe as it is today, compared to decades ago.

And we can be educated in our choice of formula, voting with our dollar for the brand that is the safest, that declares all its ingredients (GM--labeling), and so on.

Softening our attitude does not mean that we believe formula is as good as breastmilk or that we condone what the industry has done historically around the world (if you are unaware of these global issues, save your research for later, now is the time for healing).

It also does not mean that we trivialize our grief about breastfeeding not going as hoped.

Rather, it means that we accept the value and importance of formula now in our situation.

Please also take a moment to appreciate that mothers have options today which decades ago were not available:

Breastmilk donated from mothers or obtained from breastmilk-banks

Low-allergen recipes for homemade formula using organic ingredients

Organic powdered formula made with quality ingredients

Another reframe: We can truly feel grateful for the mothers and lactation experts who have gone before us, pioneering these more healthful supplemental foods.

EMOTIONALLY EMPTY AT THE PUMP

A frequent pumping schedule can feel like the straw that breaks the camel's back. "On top of everything else, now I have to pump?"

Some mothers do manage to pump long term, even pumping while commuting, and pumping at work. They might use their pumping time to read or connect online. They might watch their favorite shows. Or they might meditate, pray, or look at photos of their baby while pumping.

But for mothers experiencing breastfeeding grief, being obliged to pump and then perhaps not seeing the hoped-for result can compound feelings of grief.

Pumping also makes some mothers feel alone or diminished, and can bring up feelings of isolation, abandonment, and failure.

It is important to take these feelings seriously. Rather than pushing them away, we can breathe through them and turn our focus toward a healing thought or visualizations, as described in Part Two.

It is helpful to re-purpose our time at the pump so that it is of value to us. For instance, you could read a book, do relaxation and visualization exercises, record an oral journal, rap an improvised song over the rhythm of the pump, think about things you like and look forward to, and so on.

One of the most difficult questions that pumping mothers face is whether it would be better to spend that time with their baby. Indeed, if pumping monopolizes most of a mother's available time, and it sometimes does, especially if a mother works or cares for older children, she might very well consider whether it is better to simply spend this time with her family.

This decision is a mother's own to make. Life is not always optimal. Assessing our challenges and reaching a decision reflects our growing maturity. Finding peace with our decisions is an ongoing process.

USING A SUPPLEMENTER AT THE BREAST (SNS OR LACT-AID)

The Good News: a supplementer (a small bottle or sack with a fine tube that is taped to the nipple) allows many mothers to feed at the breast with their breastmilk, with donated breastmilk, or topped off with formula.

Feeding this way can save the breast-nurturing relationship. Even if the mother has little or no supply, there is still the physical relationship that is emotionally comforting for both. As well, the stimulation a mother receives from her baby's suckling might save her supply, even if it remains at low production.

If you do not know how to use a supplementer, or if you have questions as to which brand would be easiest to use, research online and talk to your breastfeeding mothers' group or to your lactation expert.

The Bad News: Some mothers find it hard to use a supplementer. It can feel awkward or cumbersome, and a baby will occasionally refuse to accept the tubing, try what one might.

If it doesn't work out, mothers tend to feel guilty. They check off another "failure" on the long list of "If only I'd done it differently."

It is very important to acknowledge that all of us have limits as to what we can take on at any one time. We should support each other in our processes of self-acceptance and self-forgiveness.

RETURNING TO WORK

In the United States, parents do not have the right to a paid leave of absence after childbirth, in contrast to other western countries, and US mothers return to work earlier than they would like.

Nature did not intend mothers and babies to be separated, and for some of us, the stress of work and separation from our baby affects our supply. Mothers who were struggling to make a full supply might now see it grow less. This can be heartbreaking.

Another challenge is getting enough sleep at night to be fully alert at work. Encouraging your baby to sleep through the night will remove night feedings, and can reduce your milk out-put.

Remember, if you are losing your supply, and if you cannot pump, and if you have to stop night nursing, a supplementer (see section above) at the breast can at least save the *breast nurturing* relationship.

But even if we pump at work and maintain our supply, we might still feel all the emotions of breastfeeding grief, the anger, guilt, sadness and shame, simply because we are now separated from our baby, and our heart reacts to that.

The exercises in this book, especially the anxiety-relief exercises at the beginning of Part Two, the energy bonding visualization and the visualization to help mothers with separation may help you maintain your sense of connection to your baby, and reduce feelings of sadness and grief.

PLANNING FOR NEXT TIME

When planning for another child, mothers are frequently very afraid of a repeat of their previous breastfeeding challenges. Some even say they would rather not have another child than go through the struggles again.

Mothers tend to find, however, that a second go is an opportunity to prove to themselves how much more knowledgeable, flexible, and in control of the situation they have become.

Mothers draw up plans to eat well and take herbs during pregnancy, they make sure to have herbs, a pump, a supplementer, and whatever else they might need close at hand following childbirth.

And if breastfeeding again doesn't work out, at least we know we gave it our best effort, and feel proud of that.

MEDICAL PROBLEMS THAT REQUIRE WEANING

Breastfeeding loss and grief are especially poignant for mothers who must wean for medical reasons such as chemotherapy, mastectomy, certain infectious diseases, or when medications are incompatible with breastfeeding.

It is important to be fully informed. Ask your IBCLC about your medication. She will have the latest books at hand and can go online to her professional resources to find the best information. She might be able to suggest similar medication that is safe to take while breastfeeding.

Please also know that medicine is an evolving science, and that we do not yet have all the answers. Infectious diseases such as Lyme disease and AIDS are still subjects of debate as far as recommendations for pregnancy and breastfeeding. I suggest that mothers with these and other infectious or autoimmune conditions take the initiative to review the critical literature about pregnancy, breastfeeding and medication. Also, be sure to join patient-organized self-help groups, as members of these groups are often more up-to-date with current studies than busy doctors.

Being compelled to stop breastfeeding due to medical issues might trigger feelings of anxiety, helplessness, and, in some cases, victimization. Please honor all your emotions and find the support you need to go forward.

D-MER – SUFFERING WITH THE LETDOWN REFLEX

Rarely, mothers experience a disorder known as D-MER (Dysphoric milk ejection reflex) in which difficult physical sensations and painful emotions erupt with the letdown reflex. Mothers who experience D-MER might feel nauseous or emotionally traumatized each time they pump or feed their baby, and of course they suffer all the emotions of breastfeeding grief, such as loss, despair, and anger.

If you have D-MER, the practices of relaxation and mindfulness, and the healing visualizations for heart-to-heart connection with your baby, can help you gain the sense of safety and control you need. Hypnotherapy has also proven helpful; it can help reduce the pain and nausea and speed up the perceived flow of time so the spell passes more quickly. Hypnotherapy is of special value for mothers whose D-MER emotions seem connected to their childhood.

Please educate yourself about D-MER and connect with mothers who have this problem. For information about the role of nutrition, herbs, and physical therapy such as craniosacral and chiropractic, see the website:

http://www.d-mer.org/Natrualtreatment.html

GRIEF AND ANGER

Grief and anger are somewhat like sisters--they often appear together and can be hard to tell apart. But although the intensity is similar with both, grief turns us inward, and anger turns us outward.

Anger, in some ways, is an easier emotion than grief. We may know angry, aggressive people who are apparently successful, but we rarely see successful people who are grieving. For many of us, grief is scary, unknown territory, whereas anger seems familiar. In comparison to grief, anger can feel safe.

The problem with anger after birth is that, in many cases, there is no good target for our anger. Without a target, mothers turn their anger toward the wrong people—toward themselves, toward their partners, toward their children, and even toward their baby.

Being angry can momentarily relieve some of the pent-up pressure we may feel, but anger cannot heal grief. Eventually, we have to turn toward our pain, feel it, breathe through it, and find a way to express it, through tears, creativity, writing, etc.

Below, you can read about some of the ways that grieving mothers tend to feel and express anger.

ANGRY WITH MYSELF

Grieving mothers are often angry with themselves, for instance, at their body or breasts if they believe they are the problem. Mothers then say, "My body failed me, and I just can't stand my breasts."

Mothers often blame themselves for not having prevented whatever difficulty they encountered. We say, "If I had only prepared better, read this or that book, gone to this or that class, hired a doula (or hired a different doula), chosen a different hospital, been more forceful about our birth plan," and so on.

You may be surprised to learn just how universal these thoughts and feelings are, and that countless mothers, right now as you read these words, are judging themselves harshly in precisely this way.

With time, you can use the fiery energy of anger to be productive for positive change.

ANGRY WITH BREASTFEEDING ADVOCATES

When mothers invest time and money preparing to breastfeed, by reading, going to classes, following blogs and websites, and watching breastfeeding experts on YouTube, only to discover that their own challenges were barely touched upon, they naturally feel cheated.

If this describes you, you are not alone.

Of course, mothers today have much more information and support than mothers ever had before. However, there is still a lot to do and accomplish, and the feedback of mothers like you helps move that process along.

I encourage you to speak out. Send a letter or email to the editors of a magazine or the authors of books you've read (email or slow-mail C/O the publishing house). Write the contact-person of a breastfeeding advocacy or education group.

In some cases, the authors or editors may be unaware of the issue you've dealt with. Explain your experience and the kind of information you would have needed. Express that you were disappointed not to find information and support for your issues in this resource. Your communication can help move breastfeeding advocacy in a more comprehensive direction.

ANGRY WITH MY HEALTHCARE PROVIDERS

Mothers may be angry with hospital personnel for what is known as *breastfeeding mismanagement.* This might be the case, for instance, if a nurse did not respect your wish not to bottle-feed at night; if it was the weekend and no lactation consultants were available; if a baby's tongue-tie was not diagnosed or treated properly; if you were not told about different ways to pump or hand express your milk; if you received contradictory or inadequate guidance; and so on.

If this describes you, I encourage you to write a letter or email, explaining what happened to you and expressing your dissatisfaction. If your complaint is toward an individual person such as a midwife, doula or lactation consultant, please share your complaint directly with them, per email or private message. As a rule, professionals in the birth and breastfeeding scene are doing their best in the face of enormous pressure. Yet, they can learn from the feedback of their clients. In return, they may share information with you. Hopefully, if they were in the wrong, they will extend their apologies or sympathy in a way that helps you find resolution for your anger.

If your complaint is toward the hospital or clinic, send your complaint to the appropriate department or person at the hospital. If you do not receive a satisfactory response, look online at complaints toward that hospital or clinic, and add yours to the list.

Or share your complaint with your local mothers' group, with a local newspaper, local blog, or online complaint forum. You may discover that your complaint is pushing forward changes in the hospital or clinic.

Oh no! Angry with my Baby?

To an overwhelmed, struggling mother, a baby's challenges can feel like betrayal, as if their baby is not doing their part to make breastfeeding work.

For instance, when a baby does not latch on, or does not stay latched on the breast, mothers might take it personally and feel as though their baby is "doing it wrong on purpose," choosing to reject them.

Similar feelings can arise when a baby is unable to suckle well, or is having problems digesting the mother's milk, such as with colic, GERD-reflux, food sensitivities and food allergies.

While the rational part of our mind knows that our baby's behavior has nothing to do with us personally, another, vulnerable part can easily feel rejected when our baby arches away from the breast, makes a face of disgust or pain, or screams during or after a feeding.

In spite of knowing that our newborn is not deliberately rejecting or betraying or undermining our breastfeeding efforts, the feeling of betrayal or rejection can seem very real and cause mothers tremendous emotional pain, to the extent that some mothers actually struggle with feelings of anger toward their baby.

If you are feeling anything in this direction, please realize that these unfortunate feelings are very common. Because breastfeeding is primal and instinctual, these responses rise up from parts of the brain that are not rational. It is not your fault that you feel this way.

Please get help for latch and sucking issues. Colic, GERD-reflux and food allergies can also be addressed and improved. Tongue and lip ties, which interfere with latching and a good suck, can usually be treated so that a good latch and suck are possible.

Physiological Factors that Contribute to Anger

People often think of anger, irritability, fatigue or depression as character flaws. Yet, each "flaw" often has a physiological cause that requires nutritional or medical support, and/or lifestyle changes. When the physiological cause has been addressed, the difficult "character trait" simply disappears! It wasn't a "flaw" after all!

Physiological factors that contribute to anger include:

o   Nervous exhaustion and nervous system stress

o   Premenstrual Syndrome (PMS) or Premenstrual Dysphoric Disorder (PMDD)

o   Blood sugar imbalances, insulin dysregulation

o   Fatigue, such as from low blood iron

o   Depression

o   Toxicity, liver congestion, liver pathways imbalance

o   Candidiasis (fungal infection of the intestine)

o   Mercury toxicity, such as from silver fillings in the teeth

o   Lyme disease "Lyme rage" is a common symptom of chronic Lyme disease

o   If you have anger issues or other difficult emotions that do not resolve, consider the possibility that there may be underlying, physiological causes. Start with an Internet search on each of the terms above. For more support, see a specialist who is trained in "functional medicine" (looks at root causes, rather than symptoms), a nutritionist, MD or naturopath or other. There are also many books and websites that can help you.

THE PRECIOUS CORE OF SADNESS

At some juncture on the healing journey, you might feel great sadness.

If this happens to you, don't fight it. Make room for the sadness in your chest and body. Use the breathing exercise in Part Two to be fully with it. Let the sadness flow as tears if that feels right, listen to soothing music if that feels right, talk with a friend, hug your spouse, write a poem or song, do simple things such as watering the plants, taking a walk alone, or just sit still and be with your sadness.

You see, we may not have been able to have the birth or the breastfeeding experience we looked forward to, and we may have suffered and struggled and still carry regrets about that, but we nonetheless still have all the love and nurturing within us that we need and want for our babies and ourselves.

This understanding reveals itself when we listen to our sadness and feel our way to its core.

There, like the pearl hidden in the oyster, we find our precious regard for life, and our profound desire to be in connected and healthy relationships.

If we didn't care so much, we would not feel such sadness.

It is our caring heart, hidden within our sadness, which guides our path toward healing.

Part Two

Practices to Help You Heal

Anxiety Relief Exercises

Focused Relaxation Exercises

Mindfulness Practices and Meditation

Guided Visualizations

Journal Prompts

Transforming Your Emotions

INTRODUCTION TO PART TWO

In Part Two, you will be guided through easy-to-do relaxation and emotional processes that are widely used by therapists to change the way the brain responds to stress.

These processes have been explored and applied, all the way back to the famous psychiatrist Milton Erickson, whose astonishing practice in the 1930s and 40s became a source of inspiration for later generations of therapists.

As a child, Erickson recognized the principles of hypnotherapy. He used them to heal his own body that had been paralyzed from childhood polio: he overcame his paralysis and led a normal life.

Erickson recognized that what we create, believe and "model" in our mind profoundly affects the body and emotions.

Today, the science of "neuroplasticity" is rediscovering and defining these same principles. We are discovering how our thoughts and beliefs affect processes in the body, and even the kinds of genes that are expressed in our cells, *moment to moment*.

We also know today that new cells are constantly created in the brain, and that they can form new "pathways" that hold the new thoughts and feelings we create. But when we are depressed, cell production slows down, and we are less able to learn and adapt. Still, if we practice relaxation and focus on thoughts that help us feel better (see "reframing" in Part One), our brain can again pick up its production of new cells and form pathways for better ways of feeling. *The brain can heal.*

Part Two is written in an easily understandable way. While reading or listening to it, your brain can already begin to become more adaptive and begin its deeper healing.

At healingbreastfeedinggrief.com, you can purchase a recording of Part Two, and a Journal Workbook is planned.

ANXIETY RELIEF EXERCISES

"No one ever told me that grief felt so much like fear." – C.S. Lewis

Mothers struggling to breastfeed often feel anxious.

When we feel anxious, the body responds. The muscles around the eyes tense up and the eyes appear smaller. The eyebrows scrunch together. The jaw tightens, and the muscles in the neck constrict. Our breathing is shallow, and it speeds up. There may be a feeling of pressure around the heart.

The following exercises help the body relax in very specific ways. When the body relaxes and releases these stress responses, the mind and emotions follow. We are relieved of the prior feelings of anxiety.

I recommend that you try each of these exercises separately, and then link them together in four consecutive steps. Soon, you will go through the steps in seconds, instantly switching into a calmer state of mind.

A great place to practice this is alone in the shower. As a mother of young children, the shower may soon become one of the very few places you can count on (sometimes) being alone, and mothers tell me that using this time to feel better with these simple exercises is doable and effective.

PERIPHERAL SIGHT

1) Gaze steadily in front of you. Blink a few times to relax your eyes, to "soften" your gaze. Now imagine that you are taking in more and more of everything you see around the outside, or the periphery, of your vision. Your vision becomes a little blurry as your gaze expands outwards. Your eyes relax and your gaze feels softer and softer.

2) Breathe in and out and hold this softer, expanded vision. Imagine that you can see the space above and beneath you, and behind you.

3) Now notice how you feel.

4) Perhaps you would like to adjust the position of your head. Maybe your neck has released a little of its former tension.

*

When we soften our gaze and take in our peripheral sight, we signal to the brain that we are safe. As a result, our muscles let go and we begin to breathe more slowly and deeply.

Once you have practiced this a few times, you can do the same exercise with your eyes closed. Yes, you don't have to have your eyes open to soften your gaze. Simply imagine your vision softening and expanding all around and even behind you.

You can practice this in the shower, before pumping or feeding your baby, before sleep and upon waking—anytime that you want to signal to your body and brain that all is well.

JAW RELAXATION

1) Purse your lips, tighten your jaw and clench your teeth for a second. (Don't overdo it; you don't want to crack a tooth!) Now relax, let your jaw relax and your lower jaw drop. Feel the muscles around your mouth relax as completely as possible, the large muscles and tiny muscles. You can open your mouth as your bottom jaw lowers, or keep your lips together, and let them become soft and relaxed

2) Now, with your tongue, gently moisten your lips.

*

A relaxed jaw and moist lips are indicative of a safe, relaxed state. Your brain will notice this change in your body and begin to release more feelings of anxiety. You might notice a gentle dissolving of mental tension and a lightening of your mood.

You can repeat this exercise throughout the day, for instance, in the shower, before getting up in the morning, before eating, before or while pumping or feeding your baby, and so on.

COUNTDOWN

Another way to relax is with a countdown. If you have already done the peripheral sight and jaw relaxation exercises, you can now begin counting down *on each out-breath*, silently or out loud. You can count down from ten to one, from five to one, from three to one—whichever is best for you. Again, with each exhalation, count down one number at a time, all the way to one.

Maybe you've seen a sit-com where a character counts down from ten to one in order to prevent an outburst of anger. The funny part is when the character explodes anyway. On television, this is funny, but in real life, it is not funny if we cannot find a way to shift our feelings out of stress or anger.

The trick is this: When you soften your gaze and relax your jaw and form your intention to relax, the countdown can now become a powerful way to deepen the feelings of calm and safety that you have already begun to create.

Simply by holding the intention to sink into deeper relaxation as you count yourself down with each number, you may be amazed at your transition into a much more relaxed, calm and peaceful state of mind, heart, and body. Try it!

HEART BREATHING

After doing one or more of the above exercises, close your eyes and focus on your heart. Maybe you can feel where it is in your body, and get in touch with its pumping. However much or little you can sense this is okay.

After a moment, see of you can sense what some call the "heart energy." Maybe you can feel it, and maybe instead of feeling it, you can imagine it. For some, the heart energy is in the heart. It might also be felt in the center of the chest, to one side, or further back, closer to your spine.

As a new mother, you might feel this heart-energy radiating out into your breasts, or down your arms into your hands, and even into your belly, where your baby recently lived. You might feel this, or you might imagine it. Both are good.

Perhaps you can imagine this energy as a color, such as soft pink, or soft green, or a golden color.

Now, inhale into your heart area, and exhale from your heart area. Breathe in to your heart energy, and out from your heart energy.

If you keep your focused attention on your heart energy for a minute or two, you will probably find that you are entering a more peaceful and naturally confident state.

This is a beautiful exercise to do while feeding your baby or while enjoying skin-to-skin and/or heart-to-heart time with your baby.

A FOUR STEP PRACTICE (EASY TO DO IN THE SHOWER)

Under the comfortable flow of warm water…

1) Take a moment to relax your eyes and to soften and expand your gaze.

2) Now allow your jaw to tense, and then relax your jaw. Moisten your lips.

3) On each out-breath, count yourself down into relaxation.

4) Now become aware of the heart energy in your chest, and breathe around and through your heart.

Focused Relaxation Exercises

This exercise is called focused relaxation because we both focus our attention while also allowing ourselves to relax.

You see, usually, when we focus our attention, we tend to tense up mentally and physically. And if we relax, we tend to mentally de-focus, and to drift in and out. We are accustomed to doing only one of the two: either to focus, or to relax. But here, we do both.

This leads to a feeling of wholeness, peace and comfort.

Focused Relaxation is a good preparation for each of the other exercises in Part Two, the guided visualizations, mindfulness practices, and journaling. It is also, of course, a wonderful practice to do during heart-to-heart connection with your baby.

A Recorded Version

If you would like, you can speak these instructions slowly into a recording device and listen to them while you do the exercise. Wherever you see a comma, or several dots in a row, leave a 1-3 second pause.

You can also ask someone to record the instructions. It should be a person you trust and whose voice is comforting and reassuring to you.

You may also purchase a recording of these exercises, spoken by the author, at the website www.healingbreastfeedinggreif.com.

Simple Steps to Focus-Relax

1) To begin, close your eyes. Take a deep breath, hold it for a moment . . . and then release the air in a smooth flow through your nose or your mouth. Do this two more times (in your recording, leave time for the breaths) . . . and begin to breathe naturally through your nose . . . the in-breath . . . and the out-breath . . .

2) As you bring your attention to your breath, notice that at the very end of an out-breath, you can discover a tiny pause in the natural flow of the breath . . . just when the out-breath reaches its deepest point. As you become aware of the pause at the deepest point of the out-breath . . . see if you can identify a sense of letting go . . . and a feeling of gently sinking down . . . inside yourself . . .

3) Now, you can begin counting yourself down, from ten to one . . . just having the intention to go deeper into relaxation . . . while counting your exhalations . . . allows you to settle down deeper . . . into a deep relaxed state.

4) Enjoy this relaxed state for a while. You can deepen it even more with one of the visualizations, or continue to allow yourself to go more and more deeply into relaxation with each breath.

5) When you are ready to conclude the session, say, "Next time, I will easily relax this deeply, and relax even deeper still." Take a moment to gently stretch and return to the present moment. Open your eyes.

*

Breathing techniques, relaxation suggestions and visualizations have been used therapeutically for over a hundred years.

For instance, they form the basis of neuropsychiatrist Dr. Daniel G. Amen's book, Change Your Brain, Change Your Life: The Breakthrough Program for Conquering Anxiety, Depression, Obsessiveness, Anger, and Impulsiveness. I mention Dr. Amen's book to assure the critical reader that science and clinical experience stand behind these simple breathing techniques and mental relaxation practices. They really do work.

ADVANCED VERSION

1) As you pay attention to your breath . . . notice that at the very end of the out-breath, when your lungs are empty . . . and at the very top of an in-breath, when your lungs are full . . . there is "pause" . . . a moment of stillness . . . that you can discover.

2) Like a child on a swing, there is this . . . moment of suspension . . . of weightlessness . . . before the swing changes direction . . . from the in-breath, to the out-breath, to the in-breath. As you become aware of the pause at the top of the in-breath, see if you can identify a sense of being filled . . . and at the pause at the end of the out-breath, see if you can identify a sense of letting go, a feeling of gently sinking down, possibly of discovering deep peace . . . and a feeling of safety.

PROGRAMMING ON THE OUTBREATH

1) The out-breath is a time during which whatever affirmations you say to yourself will be easily accepted and taken in by your unconscious mind.

2) For example, while breathing out slowly and gently, you can say something positive and relaxing such as "deeper and deeper relaxed," "letting go," "relaxing all the way down to my feet," or "all tension releasing."

When you lay down to sleep, you could say, "Sleep, now, sleep," on your out-breath, or count yourself down into sleep, "10, sleep... 9, sleep now sleep, 8, drifting down into sleep..." and so on.

If you only have 10 minutes to nap, you could say, "In 10 minutes, awaken fully rested..."

If you are preparing to pump, breastfeed or supplement feed, you can say, "milk gently beginning to flow," and "love flowing to my baby," or "love enveloping me and my baby."

3) When you have relaxed as much as you would like at present, conclude by saying, again on your out-breath, "Next time, I will relax this deeply and even deeper still."

If you practice focused relaxation exercises each day, you may soon be able to quickly go from feeling stress to feeling relaxation. To practice this transition, say to yourself on your out-breath, "Ten . . . One." Let your attention move like a wave over your body, from your head to your toes, flooding your body with the intention to relax.

MINDFULNESS PRACTICES AND MEDITATION

In recent years, mindfulness meditation has attracted a lot of attention. Researchers have discovered that even just one week of as little as 7 - 20 minutes a day relieves stress, improves concentration, builds empathy and compassion, and, importantly, is helpful in the treatment of posttraumatic stress syndrome.

It's no wonder that trainings in mindfulness are now given to teachers and students, to hospital staff and terminally ill patients, to Olympic athletes and Google nerds, to returning vets and to CEOs—and also to parents and children.

Mindfulness refers to awareness. It describes a focused state of mind in which we are observing our experience.

In essence, mindfulness distinguishes two parts of the mind: the part that *identifies* with the body, thoughts and feelings, and the part *observes* the body, thoughts and feelings as if from a distance. This latter part is called the "observer" or "witness."

For example, right now, you have thoughts and feelings about what you are reading. You might be enjoying these words, or they might bore you. You might be intrigued by what is described here, or you might find these concepts hard to take in and be uneasy about that.

Whatever you are thinking and feeling now, if you take a mental step back and observe your thoughts and feelings, you can begin to understand what is meant by "witness awareness."

Witness awareness can be very helpful when life seems overwhelming, as it often does for parents. Being able to pull back from difficult emotions and see the situation with a fresh perspective is one of the benefits of a mindfulness practice.

However, if we develop a detached, observing mind, we risk becoming emotionally uninvolved in our life. This is why we also bring feelings of kindness and compassion into the mindfulness practice, for instance, by imagining the breath as being warm or friendly.

As we inhale, we imagine that we are inviting a kind, warm breath into our body. If we are pregnant, we imagine this friendly breath flowing into our womb and surrounding our baby. If breastfeeding, we imagine the affectionate breath entering our heart, our chest, breasts, and of course, flowing out with the milk, even flowing down through our arms and around our baby. If bottle-feeding, we also bring this beautiful breath into our chest, breasts, arms, bottle, and baby. We allow the feeling of kindness embrace both of us.

Teachers of mindfulness call this practice "mindfulness with kindfulness."

In the next section, I will describe a beginner's mindfulness practice that you can record, and it is also available on the Healing Breastfeeding Grief website as an MP3.

A Basic Mindfulness Practice

To prepare for this practice, sit comfortably, close your eyes and relax. Begin with the anxiety-relief techniques that are described at the beginning of Part Two. Bring a sense of relaxation to your eyes, to your jaw, and count yourself into relaxation, 3, 2, and 1.

When you are ready, bring your attention to your breath—your in-breath, and your out-breath. As your breath flows in and out, notice the sensation at your nostrils, the coolness of the air entering your nostrils, and its warmth as you exhale.

Notice how, with your in-breath, your body rises a bit, and with your out-breath, how your body sinks a little, how it settles down, each time a little more, with each out-breath. And that with the flow of your breath, your head, neck and shoulders make slight adjustments, releasing tension, finding new balance and alignment.

To help keep your mind from distractions, you can begin to count your breaths down from 5 to 1, and then repeat again. Counting your breaths helps keep your focus fully in the moment.

Or you may want to repeat to yourself "Just this breath," saying "Just this" on the in-breath, and "breath" on the out-breath. Repeating "just this . . . breath" enables you to be fully present with each breath, each moment.

And you can imagine or feel how this breath has a warm quality to it. The oxygen in each breath nourishes and energizes each cell of your body. With the next in-breath, feel how the friendly warmth streams into your body, and how the warmth spreads throughout your body, more and more, with each in-breath.

At some point, you might notice that you have thoughts and feelings, coming and going. And that is perfectly normal. This is what the mind does: it creates thoughts and feels feelings. That is the mind's job. You don't have to be concerned with the thoughts or feelings. You can just notice them, and return your concentration to your friendly breath.

Thoughts and feelings might also come up that make you uncomfortable. If this happens, allow yourself to observe them, as if from a distance.

You might also visualize yourself on a green meadow and above you, a beautiful blue sky . . . and imagine that these thoughts or feelings are now a little cloud, high in the sky, floating in a high, far-away wind to the horizon. Watch the cloud move across the sky, disappearing behind the horizon, and notice that the sky is perfectly clear and blue, and your mind, still.

Return your focus to your breath.

If you practice even just a few minutes of mindfulness, now and then during the day, and as you get used to it and your mind quiets more quickly, you might notice that you can turn your attention upon itself… that your awareness can become aware of its own focused stream of attention. This is the energy of your aware mind.

Your focused awareness is naturally interested, even curious, about whatever it is focusing on. Awareness does not judge. It is interested, it observes, moment by moment, the thoughts and feelings that pass before it. It does not try to change anything.

Now, if you are feeding your baby, your attention can focus on this experience, on sensations such as the pressure of your body where you sit or lie, on the sensations of muscles that are active or tense as you hold your baby, and as you focus on your muscles, they automatically become a little more relaxed. And you can be aware of the feeling of your baby close to you, your shared warmth, and hear the sounds of your baby swallowing, or the weight of your sleeping baby, sensing your baby's calm breathing.

Feel yourself, feel your baby, present and calm.

As you do this practice, your breathing will be slowing, your brainwaves becoming smoother, your body is better oxygenated, and you feel more relaxed. Your baby will be sensing and enjoying all these subtle changes, too. Your baby senses the gentle quality of your attention, the open friendliness of your heart, and the comfort of your presence.

After this mindfulness practice, you can go on if you would like to the "envelop your baby with love" visualization, or heart-to-heart connection, or your own preferred meditation, visualization or prayer.

Remember, the part of us that is "focused relaxed" is never bored or tired. It is interested, even curious. There is a quality of joy within it. Aliveness.

Now and then, during these practices, you might become conscious of your awareness, of the light of your mind.

While aware of your awareness, let the comfortable heaviness of your body act as an anchor, so that when beautiful sensations begin to fill you, you remain grounded in your body. Imagine that you can breathe these beautiful feelings into and throughout your body and mind.

EMOTIONAL HEALING WITH MINDFULNESS

Mindfulness meditation can support emotional healing. It gives us the ability to simply "be" with our feelings. It calms the urge to judge or change our feelings. We become less reactive, and no longer push our feelings down or away.

When we simply breathe through our emotions in a nonjudgmental way, our emotions surprise us by beginning to lighten and change. The healing that occurs when people do this simple practice has amazed researchers, and you will hopefully be amazed, too.

GUIDED VISUALIZATIONS

In traditional societies around the world, mothers are given a little vacation, or time-off from life, in the month after childbirth. Not only are mothers are fed and massaged; others also take over the work in her house or garden. Even shopping and cooking are done for her. This supportive "team" cocoons a mother, so that she can fully focus on her baby and emerge as a strong, healthy and happy mother.

But there's more. Having loving, helpful persons around us after childbirth can serve as a "model" for the behavior of mothering. You see, our brains learn by observation and imitation. We mimic the behavior we see, until it is securely our own. "Modeling" is how we learned how to talk, walk, play and behave when we were little, and it is also how we learn to be a mother.

If your nurse, doula or lactation consultant was good at her job, she will have shown you some initial mother-modeling. She will have spoken kindly to you, smiled warmly at your baby while exuding sweet admiration, and she will have told you what a beautiful baby you've brought into this world. With such positive modeling, our healthcare team helps us feel good about motherhood.

Indeed, if your nurse or lactation consultant was warm and confident, you might have found breastfeeding to be easier as long as she was present, even that your baby latched onto your breast more securely and that your milk flowed more abundantly as long as she was nearby. It may have also been easier to connect with your baby emotionally and to feel good and hopeful about being a parent. This is what being close to a good mothering model can do for us.

Unfortunately, in our modern world, mothers do not receive much support or extra care in the weeks after childbirth. Just the opposite: we often feel as though *we* are supposed act as a hostess for visiting friends or family. Sometimes, mothers feel all alone, as if in a vacuum, with our own needs.

For many mothers, breastfeeding groups are the only source of modeling. Some mothers in these groups have been through the hoops and matured in their mothering skills—including having a generous heart for new mothers. Just being together with secure and knowledgeable mothers can be so reassuring. Even if you are not nursing, it can feel good to participate in a local breastfeeding or mothering group, simply for the community and modeling that all of us need.

The good news is that through the practice of guided visualization and hypnotherapy, we can also receive some of this positive, cocooning mother-modeling. We can, for instance, visualize times and places in which we felt secure, happy, and confident. We can visualize people who let us feel that we are deeply loved, valued, and accepted, such as a dear friend, or favorite aunt or grandmother who represents secure warm love. And if we did not experience such times and places in our life, and if we did not have supportive persons in our life, we can make them up. We can simply imagine what it would feel like to be in such a great place, and with a supportive person. That works, too. The brain takes in the visualization as though it was really happening, and we imbue our mother-self with confidence, security, love, trust and honor.

VISUALIZATION ONE: SAFE PLACE

To prepare for this practice, sit comfortably, close your eyes and relax. Begin with the anxiety-relief techniques. Bring a sense of relaxation to your eyes, to your jaw, and count yourself into relaxation, 3, 2, 1.

When you are ready, bring your attention to your breath; your in-breath, and your out-breath. As your breath flows in and out, notice the sensation at your nostrils, the coolness of the air entering your nostrils, and its warmth as you exhale.

Notice how, with your in-breath, your body rises a bit, and with your out-breath, your body sinks a little, settles down, with each out-breath it relaxes more deeply, and that with the flow of your in-breath, and your out-breath, your head, neck and shoulders make slight adjustments, releasing tension, finding new balance and alignment.

Now I invite you to imagine a beautiful safe place. Perhaps it is somewhere you've been on vacation, a place you know where you can deeply relax, or it is a favorite room where you feel warm and cozy, or a beautiful garden, or simply a place that you like to imagine now. As you imagine, sense or see the details of your special place, go to a place here to sit or lie, and feel the comfortable pull of gravity on your body. Take in the details of this place, the colors, smells, sounds, feelings, and the touch of the air on your face.

Take a moment to notice the feelings you have here in your special place. Perhaps you feel comfort. Ease. Safety. Pleasure. Wonderment.

Turn your attention to your breath, and imagine that you can breathe these feelings into your body. They enter your lungs, your heart and bloodstream, and fill your body from the top of your head to the soles of your feet. They enter your bones. You can feel these good feelings in your arms, your legs, your belly, and womb.

After a while, if you notice anything that does not serve you, a feeling, thought, or something in your safe place that you would like to have gone, you can let it go with your exhalation.

Feel again your good feelings, and imagine bringing these good feelings to your life now, to yourself, and to your baby.

Take a moment to imagine some times in the future, times when you might like to find these positive feelings waiting for you—such as when feeding your baby at night, or when your baby cries—and other times when it would be helpful to find these feelings there waiting for you, and you can let these scenes pass before your mind's eye, seeing how good you feel, even in these situations, with these feelings from your special place, and allowing yourself to fully feel this.

Stay here for a while. Return to your normal consciousness whenever you like. The experiences you have here will travel with you.

Visualization Two: Loving Companion

To prepare for this practice, sit comfortably, close your eyes and relax. Begin with the anxiety-relief techniques. Bring a sense of relaxation to your eyes, to your jaw, and count yourself into relaxation, 3, 2, 1.

When you are ready, bring your attention to your breath; your in-breath, and your out-breath. As your breath flows in and out, notice the sensation at your nostrils, the coolness of the air entering your nostrils, and its warmth as you exhale.

Notice how, with your in-breath, your body rises a bit, and with your out-breath, your body sinks a little, settles down, with each out-breath it relaxes more deeply, and that with the flow of your in-breath, and your out-breath, your head, neck and shoulders make slight adjustments, releasing tension, finding new balance and alignment.

Now I invite you to imagine a beautiful safe place. Perhaps it is somewhere you've been on vacation, a place you know where you can deeply relax, or it is a favorite room where you feel warm and cozy, or a beautiful garden, or simply a place that you like to imagine now. As you imagine, sense or see the details of your special place, go to a place here to sit or lie, and feel the comfortable pull of gravity on your body. Take in the details of this place, the colors, smells, sounds, feelings, and the touch of the air on your face.

Take a moment to notice the feelings you have here in your special place. Perhaps you feel comfort. Ease. Safety. Pleasure. Wonderment.

Now I invite you to receive a visit from a safe and supportive person. Look off into the distance, and see your loving person approach.

Perhaps, as the figure comes closer, you recognize a person you feel a special connection to, may a teacher, or mentor, someone you look up to, or a dear friend. Or it might be someone you do not personally know but would have liked to know, someone you have always admired or felt a connection to.

And as that person draws close to you, you feel their presence, their closeness, and you feel the connection between you. As you look into their eyes, you feel deeply known, understood, accepted, and loved.

And anything else that you would like to feel in this connection, let it come to you now.

Take a moment to notice the beautiful feelings you have.

Now take these beautiful feelings into your body with your inhalation. The knowing, the connectedness, the love, are carried on your breath into your heart, and they flow throughout your body, entering every cell.

And anything that does not serve you, you can let go of, with your exhalation.

As your body and mind are filled with these good feelings, imagine bringing these feelings to your situation now, to yourself and to your baby.

Take a moment to imagine times when you might like to find these positive feelings waiting for you, and you can let these scenes pass before your mind's eye, and allow yourself to fully feel this—how good it will be to have these good feelings waiting for you when you need them.

Stay with this for a while, and return to your normal consciousness whenever you like. The positive experiences you have here will travel with you.

VISUALIZATION THREE: WRAP YOUR BABY WITH LOVE

Have you ever seen a mother hold her baby with such heartfelt intent that it seemed as though all the loving forces in nature were right there, enclosing or wrapping her and her baby in an aura of love?

The first time I saw this was when a very motherly friend took my young infant son into her arms. Cradled in her warm-hearted embrace, he seemed both deeply calmed and magically transported. The room seemed to vibrate with love.

I wanted to be able to do that!

I asked her about it and it turned out it was a skill she had learned, and that she could tell me the secret: she cultivated a sense of enclosure. My friend believes that when holding a baby, we can mentally tap into a feeling of being wrapped and protected, as though in a safe, warm cave, or within a sphere, or womb, of layered, vital, nourishing feelings.

The following guided visualization is based on her description. It is a wonderful visualization to practice while feeding, holding, comforting or reading a book to your baby or toddler.

Just imagine yourself and your child in a warm, protected cave, or imagine you are sitting in a favorite comfy room by a fireplace, or you might like to imagine yourself surrounded by peaceful starlight or a color that signifies comfort and safety to you. In effect, you are imagining a loving "space" within which you and your child feel gently held and loved.

One way to get in contact with these feelings is to wrap yourself in a blanket or sheet while holding or feeding your baby. You might even cover your head with a corner of the blanket. With this layer around you, you can tune into how you feel enclosed, protected and calm. In essence, you are replicating how your baby felt in your womb, and then giving that feeling to yourself and your baby.

*

To prepare for this practice, sit comfortably, close your eyes and relax. Begin with the anxiety-relief techniques. Bring a sense of relaxation to your eyes, to your jaw, and count yourself into relaxation, 3, 2, 1.

When you are ready, bring your attention to your breath; your in-breath, and your out-breath. As your breath flows in and out, notice the sensation at your nostrils, the coolness of the air entering your nostrils, and its warmth as you exhale.

Notice how, with your in-breath, your body rises a bit, and with your out-breath, your body sinks a little, settles down, with each out-breath it relaxes more deeply, and that with the flow of your in-breath, and your out-breath, your head, neck and shoulders make slight adjustments, releasing tension, finding new balance and alignment.

Feel the support of the surface beneath you. Feel the air on your cheek.

Now become aware of the space around you: Feel the space above you. Feel the space beneath you. Feel the space to your right, to your left, behind you, before you.

Now imagine that all around you is a sphere or ball of loving energy. If you would like, you can imagine a golden white light filling this sphere. This light is a source of protective, supportive, loving energy for you.

In a moment, you can imagine this light-energy concentrating above your head. Imagining this energy above your head now, and then flowing into your body through the top of your head.

As it descends down through your body in gentle golden waves, it brings deep soothing relief to all your muscles.

As the light circulates through you, it encircles your womb and your belly, and it encircles your heart, flows into your breasts, into the glands in your breasts, bringing warmth.

If you are feeding your baby now, you can imagine this light flowing out into your baby. See your baby's energy sphere filling with this energy, your baby's heart surrounded with light, and then the light flowing back from your baby into your own body, and circling your heart. And flowing again into your baby, filling your baby's body, circling your baby's heart, and flowing back to you . . . and back and forth, as long as you like.

As you engage more in this visualization, you can discover all the pathways that this loving energy finds to flow between you and your baby, and around you and your baby. For instance, with your out-breath, you can follow the heart-energy as it flows from your heart into your hands, and back into your heart with your in-breath. As it flows into your arms and hands, it also flows into your baby.

As you get a feeling for this flow, back and forth, between you, around you—your heart and your baby's heart are connected in the joyful knowing that you are together, now, and that love and nourishment are one.

JOURNALING PROMPTS

Journaling is a valuable tool. It brings us more clarity into what we are feeling and, by putting it into words, lifts some of the weight from our heart.

Because mothers are very time-pressed, I have developed a set of prompts to help you.

With these prompts you will learn a lot about yourself and you will also have a record that you can refer to in the future, to show how far you have come.

Further, your answers to these prompts will be helpful when you work through the "Transformational Question Sets" at the end of Part Two.

First, Check In — Find Your Positive Emotions

Take a moment to ask yourself two important questions:

What do I love about being a mother?

What do I love about my baby?

Find at least five answers to each question.

If you would like, you can begin your journal by answering these two important questions.

If you feel as though you need to process other emotions first, you can wait for a later time when it feels easier to focus on these questions. I'll remind you later to answer them.

Prompt One: Identify Your Difficult Emotions

Below, you will find a list of emotions that are frequently experienced by mothers whose breastfeeding did not go as hoped.

Each main emotion is listed with similar but not identical emotions. Identify the emotions that most closely describe your experience, and write them in your journal.

Then ask yourself, on a scale of 1 to 10, with 10 being the strongest, how strong is this emotion? Write that number next to the emotion.

Example:

Sadness (8)

If you identify emotions that are not listed here, add them to your journal, along with a number that rates their intensity for you today.

Examples of Emotions

1. Grief, Sadness, Sorrow

2. Fear, Anxiety, Helplessness

3. Loss, Abandonment, Desperation

4. Guilt, Shame, Remorse

5. Anger, Rage, Hate

6. Inferiority, Lack of Confidence

7. Failure, Self-blame, Self-hatred

8. Numbness, Detachment, Dissociation

PROMPT TWO: IDENTIFY TRIGGERS FOR YOUR EMOTIONS

A trigger means, simply, that a certain thought or memory of a certain situation triggers or intensifies the painful emotion.

Before beginning this exercise, do a relaxation practice to help quiet your mind and allow you to feel less anxiety.

This exercise has four steps.

1. First write down one of the strongest emotions that you identified.

2. Now close your eyes and think about the last time you felt this way. Be concrete. Where were you, what did you look like, what did you see and hear? Just thinking about and remembering this situation will make the feeling much clearer and stronger. Perhaps you can look a little deeper and find one or two more triggers for this emotion by remembering other times you have felt this way.

3. Now write down the triggers you discovered.

4. Next to each trigger, write a number between 1 and 10 to show how intense the feelings are that that trigger evokes.

For example:

Sadness. For the feared loss of bonding (10), for not having to supplement with formula (10), when I think about my disappointed breastfeeding dreams (8)

Just work through one or two of the main emotions in the beginning. Later, as needed, you can work through more. It depends upon you, on how you feel, on how much time you have, and on how comfortable you are with this process.

PROMPT THREE: DISCOVER MORE CONCRETE DETAILS

This exercise is optional. If it is difficult or painful, skip it and go on to the next section.

Reverse the prompt. To do this, focus on a specific trigger (event, challenge, experience) and note which emotion or combination of emotions come up for you. Note their intensity.

The exercise is done in three steps:

1. Write down the trigger you've identified (challenge, event or experience).

2. Close your eyes, breathe in and out a few times (the relaxation practice), and then feel your way into the emotions associated with that experience. Write them down.

3. Mark the emotions on a scale of one to ten to show which ones are strongest or weakest in the mix.

For example:

My Trigger: I gave birth on a Friday night, and did not see a lactation consultant while in hospital because they are not available on weekends.

My emotions with this are: anger (10), despair (4), sadness (8), helplessness (7)

Here is a sample list of challenges. Please journal any additional triggers you discover for yourself that are not listed here, find the associated emotions, and rate them numerically. And while this book focuses on breastfeeding, if you have painful emotions associated with your pregnancy or birth experience, you can include these in this journaling process as well.

TRIGGERS (CHALLENGES, EVENTS, EXPERIENCES)

o   Medical conditions, yours or your baby's

o   Mismanagement at hospital sets you up for breastfeeding problems or failure (bottle feeding, forcefully pushing the baby on the breast, separation from mother)

o   Baby is born on a weekend or holiday, and qualified lactation experts are not available

o   Unresolved nipple pain (usually related to problems with a baby's latching)

o   Recurrent or severe mastitis (breast infection)

o   Baby's tongue-tie and lip-tie that are undiagnosed or improperly treated

o   Baby's colic, GERD-reflux or food allergies that appear related to what mother eats

o   Depression after birth, caused by hormones or other issues that are not directly related to breastfeeding

o   Low milk supply

o   High milk supply

o   Overactive letdown reflex

o   Baby's refusing the breast

o   Lack of understanding and compassion from family, friends or healthcare providers o A feeling of, "Why didn't anyone tell me this could happen? Why wasn't I prepared?"

o In addition, other challenges can play a role, such as:

o Ambivalence around pregnancy and birth

o Social pressures around nursing in front of certain people or in public

o Fears about motherhood, concerning responsibilities, lack of freedom, etc.

o Having conflicting feelings about mothering due to one's experience with one's own mother

o Sexual abuse coming up as memory or re-traumatization during birth or breastfeeding

o A difficult relationship with the child's father, partner or spouse

o Negative attitudes of one's parents or in-laws

o A stressful work environment or having to return to work soon after birth, before feeling emotionally or physically ready

o Isolation from the attachment parenting community

CHECK IN – HAVE YOU WRITTEN DOWN YOUR POSITIVE EMOTIONS AROUND MOTHERING?

At the beginning of this section on journaling, it was recommended that you take a moment to ask yourself these two important questions:

What do I love about being a mother?

What do I love about my baby?

Find at least five answers to each question.

The answers make you feel happy and positive.

These answers are key to the transformational questions below.

TRANSFORMING YOUR EMOTIONS

Now that you have become clearer about your emotions, and you have named them and discovered their causes and triggers, you can use sets of transformational questions to lighten, release, and transform your emotions.

A Brief Explanation

This method changes the way the brain holds emotions. It is based on the science of neuroplasticity, which has been extensively studied.

Neuroplasticity tells us that "brain cells that fire together, wire together." If you can consistently fire off brain cells in new and positive ways, and if you can patch over positive feelings to your original triggers, your brain can be thoroughly wired for the new positive state.

Neuroplasticity-based exercises are ideal for new mothers for three reasons:

1) They are easy to do.

2) The answers always come from inside of you.

3) The exercises can enduringly change the way we feel, and relatively quickly, too—perfect for the new mother who is pressed for time.

Here is how it works: The following questions promote somatic awareness. That is, they enable you to feel or sense your emotion directly within your body via your intuition and imagination, rather than mentally, through your thoughts and interpretations.

First, tune in to your emotion as a set of bodily sensations and images. Then imagine or sense how these bodily sensations and images change into more positive states. For instance, if you can first imagine a painful emotion in your body as a feeling of sticky tar, begin by imagining small changes, such as a change in color, or in consistency. Use your imagination to change how the emotion looks, feels, smells or weighs in your body. Eventually, you should find that the emotion has become very light and is no longer oppressive.

Here is the key: Your brain records these internal, imagined changes as though they are actual life events that are just as real as the event that caused you to have felt badly. Your brain will now memorize this new pattern and begin to repeat it, to automatize it. As you continue to practice this exercise, your brain not only learns how to move toward the positive emotion you desire, it also begins to spread the positive state into other areas of your life.

This "re-wiring" can be so profound that people find it difficult afterwards to remember what the previous, difficult or painful state was like.

Musicians and athletic performers pay hypnotherapists and coaches thousands of dollars to rewire their brain for peak performance. There's no reason that mothers should not have access to the same methods.

TRANSFORMATIONAL QUESTION SETS

Always take a few minutes before each of these exercises to relax, to be aware of your breath and bring relaxation to your body and mind by counting down from 10 to 1.

When you are ready, open your eyes and read through the questions, taking time to feel and sense your way into the sensations in your body as you do.

When you complete the exercise, if you have time, write down your experience in your journal. Be sure to mention how you felt at the beginning of the session, and how you feel at its conclusion.

SET ONE – BASIC SOMATIC AWARENESS

In this exercise, we are never judging the feelings we have, but are simply learning how to be with them, to allow our inner attention, interest and curiosity to take note of what they do, how they feel, how they change.

1) Name a strong trigger and its strongest emotion. Ask yourself:

2) Where do I feel this emotion in my body? (If you would like, you can take some deep breaths now into that   sensation in your body, and allow it to come more clearly to your mind.)

3) If I were to give this emotion a color, a texture, a sound, what would these be?

4) Does it have motion, a kind of movement?

5) As I tune in to the emotion for a minute or two—give it at least two minutes—how does the feeling change?

6) Is it lighter or heavier? Softer or sharper? Does its color change? Its texture? Its weight?

7) Does it change into a new or different feeling?

8) Stay with this new feeling, too, for at least two minutes, while again bringing your attention to your breath, and breathing into the sensations of this feeling in your body. It, too will gradually change. At first, if you are dealing with particularly difficult feelings, the changes may be small, but from day to day, the improvement in your feelings will be quite noticeable.

There are no right or wrong answers or results to this exercise. The simple practice of staying with your emotions this way, of concentrating on physical sensations (where it is in my body, how it feels in my body) and images (what color is it, how does it move), will allow your brain to begin to access the emotional states differently.

You will see the emotions begin to lighten from day to day.

Set Two — Somatic Transformation

1) Name your trigger and the emotion it evokes.

2) Make the emotion really strong, see if you can bring it in more fully—at least a 7 on a scale of 1 to 10.

3) Ask: Where do I feel this emotion in my body?

4) Does it have weight, density, motion, color, a texture, sound?

5) Ask: what would I like to feel instead? It may be hard at first to imagine what you would prefer to feel, but stay with it.

This is the appropriate place to bring in your positive emotions around mothering--what you love about mothering, what you love about your baby. Bring in some of those feelings, bring them into your body.

6) Now take a moment to fully imagine, what would the preferred emotion feel like in your body? (Where it is in your body, its density, weight, motion, color, and so on.)

7) Stay with this new feeling—become more and more aware of its qualities. For instance, how does it change the way you sit, breathe, feel?

8) Think of situations where you would like to feel this way, and imagine yourself feeling this way in those situations, and how feeling this way makes those situations better for you. Imagine at least three situations.

9) When you feel the new emotion strongly, and you've imagined several situations with the new feeling, think of the original trigger and imagine it far away, like a picture hanging on a wall in a far corner. Perhaps, the trigger no longer brings up the old feeling, or if it does, the old feeling is now lighter.

10) OK, now focus again on the new positive feeling in your body, and make it strong again. As you do, imagine more things you might do, new ways you might act, with the new feeling in your body.

11) Think of more and more things you would look forward to in your life with this new feeling.

12) Write three things you look forward to in your journal.

Because you are a mom, feeding and holding your baby will give you periods of time when you can return to these transformative questions and emotional processing exercises.

Remember to alternate them with simple relaxation exercises, and with heart-to-heart connection practices.

Work through Sets One and Two several times before proceeding to Set Three.

SET THREE – BRING BETTER FEELINGS TO YOUR LIFE

This Set is a prompt to work through residual or new negative emotions.

1) Ask yourself: In my day-to-day life now, what situation or thought still triggers the negative emotion?

2) Now ask yourself: What would I like to feel instead?

3) Describe the preferred feeling in detail. You can journal the details if you would like.

4) Now, do the relaxed focus exercise, and count yourself down into relaxation.

5) Now imagine waking up in the morning and having your preferred feeling. Imagine what it would feel like in your body. Go into as much detail as possible. Imagine this feeling as a sensation, as a color, sound, and movement.

6) As you continue to imagine and feel this good feeling in full detail, imagine the trigger event, and imagine yourself responding to it with the new emotion in place. How do you feel different about yourself and about the trigger?

SET FOUR – HEALING YOUR INNER CHILD-SELF

Difficult emotions often have their origins in experiences that we had as children. Healing our "inner child-self" entails bringing love and protection to that part of us that still lives in us as a child. This is called "Inner Child Work.

Teal Swan, who endured profound emotional injuries during childhood, wrote about her healing in the book Shadows Before Dawn. She writes, "I was actually afraid of my childhood self at first. When I would mentally go to connect with my childhood self, I was too afraid of her to touch her. I'd have to imagine angels or warrior princesses rescuing her from the memories that she was stuck in and comforting her. Over time, I did gain the confidence to imagine myself holding my childhood self. I began to connect with my own inner child, and I began to love her. I now think that inner-child work is perhaps the very best emotional healing technique that has ever been discovered."

Here is a simple guideline to do inner child work on your own.

1) Think about the negative emotion. Feel it in your body. Make it strong.

2) Ask: When is the most recent time that I felt this emotion? Take a moment to remember.

3) Then ask yourself: When is the first time in my life that I felt this emotion?

4) Let the answer come to you by itself. See yourself as a younger person in that situation, feeling what you felt.

5) Now ask: What would I have needed back then, to feel better?

6) Imagine going back into that situation as your present, grown-up self, and giving your child-self whatever it is that you would have needed to feel better, safer, and happier. Perhaps it is some information or advice; perhaps it is protection, or a loving embrace. Perhaps your child-self needed to be taken away from a situation and brought somewhere safe or comfortable, and you can imagine yourself doing that. Or perhaps you just

need to tell your inner child that she is good, and that whatever happened was not her fault. Whatever it is, give that thing to your inner child now.

7) If you would like, you can continue by imagining yourself growing up, having received this thing that you needed. See yourself going through all the stages of your life and finally arriving at your present age, with that thing you needed securely within you today.

BREASTFEEDING AS INNER CHILD WORK

A dear friend of mine, now in her 70s, offered her experience for this book.

"One of the greatest revelations of my ability to nurse my daughter was that I could heal my own inner child so much through my love of her. As I experienced myself in the role of the loving mother I longed for but never had, my feelings of loss and abandonment were relieved, and I could begin to heal. Actually, it's a lifetime of healing. Here she is, almost 40, and by continuing to be the mother I was deprived of, I'm still healing that primary wound."

Part Three

Interviews, Stories

INTRODUCTION TO PART THREE

Who are the people who work so hard to support us?

Which challenges do they face, and what motivates these practitioners to devote themselves to the care of mothers and babies?

It occurred to me as I thought about writing this book that it would be helpful for mothers to have answers to these questions.

For each contribution in this section, I asked four questions:

o   What do you do?

o   Do you have a personal or professional experience with breastfeeding grief?

o   How do you help mothers who are experiencing breastfeeding problems and grief?

o   If you could speak to my readers, from the point of view of your life and profession, what would you say?

While a few of the contributions were made as brief email replies, most were lengthy in-person interviews. In each case, the professional shares in a personal way about their experience, motivation and work.

At the end of the book, you will find contributions from mothers who opened their hearts to share their journey through breastfeeding grief with you. I am very grateful to these mothers, thank you Bekki and Cindy!

LAURA ROE, MIDWIFE OF ASHLAND, OREGON

Laura Roe is a mother, wife and midwife. She has a BSW, MED in social work and education, and an LDM and CPM Oregon licensures for home-based midwifery. Laura has attended births for twenty-four years. She says that she sees many more breastfeeding problems today than when she began her practice.

Hilary: Do you have a personal experience around breastfeeding grief?

Laura: Yes. My first personal experience is that as a baby, I was not breastfed myself. As a young adult, I came to understand how that had impacted me. And so, through my own grief and healing, I became motivated to create a different situation for myself and my children, and to facilitate that for other mother-baby dyads.

My second experience was with my first child. No one could tell me why he wasn't gaining weight. After weeks of trying, my doctor and midwife concluded that I must not have enough milk.

But then my baby received a homeopathic remedy, and immediately and rapidly began to put on weight. I had just begun my training in midwifery, and this personal experience, which was so astonishing, so completely out-of-the-box, made me want to learn more about potential breastfeeding issues for mothers and babies, and also about complimentary medicine.

Hilary: As a midwife, how do you support mothers having breastfeeding problems?

Laura: First, I stay alert. If I can anticipate issues early on, they are less likely to reach a crisis. Nutrition, homeopathy and acupuncture are tools that I use a lot. For instance, when there's been excessive blood loss, which can impact a mother's supply, acupuncture works brilliantly for that.

For me, the larger piece around breastfeeding however is this: nature designed pregnancy and birth so that a baby can easily latch on and breastfeed after birth. When the birth process is interrupted, we see greater problems in the breastfeeding relationship. So for me, our increasing problems with breastfeeding are largely a reflection of our problems with birth.

We have an amazing craniosacral therapist in town. She is very talented. I always want her to see a baby in the first three days, even before the milk comes in. I find this work helps the baby settle into its body, and that the baby is then more able and ready to start their journey in life, and to commit to breastfeeding.

I definitely have seen many mom-baby duos that would have had breastfeeding problems if they had not seen a craniosacral specialist. Even if parents don't believe in this kind of therapy, they always notice the difference, how their baby is immediately content, more settled and relaxed.

I also find nutrition very important. What a mother eats affects her milk supply. But you know that—you wrote the book!

Hilary: Laura, what message would you like to communicate to the readers of this book?

Laura: Skin-on-skin! We know it is the start of healing, the start of bonding, the start of everything. But while that is easy to say, for many mothers, it is not easy to do.

I always tell mothers, "The time that you spend naked skin-to-skin at home in bed with your baby, realistically, is going to feel like a lot more time than you want to spend. Much more than you want."

From my point of view, healing breastfeeding grief is about more than nutrition, it is about healing the emotional bonding issues of people-to-people connections. As a society, we have become afraid of the deepest intimacy, of that profound bond . . . between a mother and her child.

But that's what we're learning now, as a community, how to truly support one another. Mothers are learning to ask for help. Friends and families are understanding the importance of bringing food and meals, and are offering help with shopping and cleaning. We are learning that moms should stay in bed with their baby, they should just stay in bed doing skin-on-skin and allow themselves to be supported, allow themselves to receive the food and help they need so they can heal that wound of intimacy in their own life and family. This is a positive change that I see.

So I would like to say to moms, be open and receptive to support from your community, a community that is learning, along with you, how to support mothers who are going through all kinds of challenges. Reach out for that support, and open yourself to receive it.

JUDITH SANFORD, CRANIOSACRAL THERAPIST
BRINGING RELIEF TO FAMILIES WHEN MOST NEEDED

Licensed Massage Therapist, Craniosacral Therapist

www.judithsanfordcranial.com

I have been practicing Craniosacral Therapy since 1991. In 2000, I added a pediatric specialty and have been blessed since then to do many hours of hands-on care for moms, babies, dads and siblings.

Craniosacral therapy works via the body's fluids. The body is circulated with many kinds of fluid—blood, lymph, cerebral spinal fluid—which bathe, nourish and support the life cycle of every cell. When we think of physical therapy, we usually think of bones, muscle and tendons. It can be a stretch for people to realize that therapy that focuses on the body's fluids can also affect muscles, bones and tendons. Craniosacral can relieve compressions in tissues and joints, can free the organs, nerves, vessels, brain, and also the breast, so that these can function optimally.

In pure cranial work, the hands are very still and the internal rhythms do the work. While some people find it hard to accept that such gentle work is "real" or has any effect, the results speak for themselves in the great majority of cases.

Ms. Sanford's Story

I was a VBAC birth. My mother had so many anesthetics that nursing never was successful. I always knew she loved me to bits, but of course, I carried scars from my birth.

Over the course of my life, I have been able to heal many of my feelings of loss through receiving massage and craniosacral therapy. Through my own work with families, I pass on the blessings I received.

The main lesson I take from all of it is this: Trust life! We are programmed for healing.

Helping Moms and Babies in the Early Postpartum

Pregnancy and birth—both natural birth and Cesarean birth—exert many pressures on the mother and baby that can slow down the dynamics of the body's fluid.

For nursing babies, cranial work can help with latching, with the suck reflex, with the baby's ability to turn her head to both sides, and with settling, sleeping, and bonding.

For the mother, cranial work, (along with the lymph drainage work that I also provide), can relieve breast congestion, help the flow of milk open up, and relieve pain that can be interfering with the let-down.

Helping each of you settle comfortably into yourself so you can be deeply present is one of the best gifts of this work. Often, both the parents and I can feel how the baby fully "arrives" into their body during a session, as the baby notices, "This is the comfortable place I want to be," and settles in.

Ms. Sanford's message to mothers experiencing breastfeeding grief

Birth is a momentous and life changing event. Optimally, the mother's body is able to work through the strong emotions, tension or physical trauma. When this doesn't occur, the mother can feel stuck, as if "out of body," unable to be fully present.

If you are depressed, these blocks are very likely part of the problem. The work of a craniosacral therapist can help relieve these blocks.

I hope you'll try it. I feel so strongly about its benefits that I offer one free home visit to all newborns and families in the first three months after birth. The sooner the better! Many other practitioners do the same, or offer low cost care for infants. Don't be afraid to ask. In can change the trajectory of all your lives.

DR. BARI HARTLEY, CHIROPRACTIC SUPPORT FOR MOTHER AND BABY THROUGHOUT PREGNANCY AND AFTER BIRTH

Chiropractor (Ph.D.), Pediatric Chiropractor

www.lifeoflovechiropractic.com

My name is Dr. Bari Hartley and I am a chiropractor who specializes in pregnancy, perinatal, and pediatric chiropractic care. I was inspired to work with families due to my understanding that our uterine environment, our birth process, and our experiences of the world as children shape who we are, how we experience the world, and ultimately the societal climate. If we can experience and interpret the world with greater ease and love from an early age, we fare better as individuals and as a human species.

A bit of history: I earned my BS in Biochemistry from Binghamton University in 2003, and chose a doctorate degree in chiropractic. After a rigorous course of study and community-based internships in pediatrics/pregnancy/postnatal care, I graduated from Northwestern College of Chiropractic in 2006. I then completed a year-long course of study with the International Chiropractic Pediatric Association that focused on the health and treatment of pregnant women and their children. I am certified in the Webster Technique, which aims to restore optimal pelvic positioning for birth, and have taken extended coursework in the Craniosacral care of infants.

It is my honor to support women in the journey to motherhood, and to make a baby's transition from uterine to outside world as gentle as possible. To foster a peaceful, healthy start for all, I provide free newborn chiropractic checks at home to the mamas I have worked with during pregnancy.

Some of the most regular concerns I encounter during these home visits relate to challenges in breastfeeding and the emotions that accompany that. While chiropractic care for baby and/or mom can help clear many of these issues, I am thankful that there are other skilled practitioners, communities of wise women and mothers, and also this loving resource by Hilary Jacobson, in cases where other guidance is needed.

While most families have heard of chiropractic, many are unaware of how it supports natural health and normal body function. Chiropractic honors the body's innate intelligence. This is the same force that created you from two cells, that helps you grow, that heals you, and maintains you in health.

This intelligence communicates through your nervous system; it coordinates every bodily function, perceives the world around you, and interprets messages from inside your body. If this communication is compromised by physical, chemical, or emotional blockages, the body's natural wellness will be affected.

Chiropractors aim to restore and maintain health naturally by providing balance to the nervous system and removing any interference to its function. Most chiropractors work with restoring normal movement to the spine to ensure that the nerves are not being affected where they exit from the spinal column. Factors like intrauterine position/constraint, the birth process itself (whether vaginal or Cesarean), physical traumas, repetitive stress, and overload of chemical or emotional stress can alter the structure of the spine/body and affect neural health in babies and mothers alike.

These spinal alterations can be gently corrected as soon after birth as a family desires. In fact, many pregnancy and pediatric focused chiropractors start their work with baby during pregnancy, by establishing balance in mom's spine and pelvis. This promotes greater health for mom, unrestricted development for the baby, and an easier birth process. In addition to working with the spine, many pediatric chiropractors also work to establish balance in the cranium (bones of the skull) soon after birth, as these are under important but varying and often uneven pressure during a vaginal birth process.

Bringing ease to mom's body (physically, neurologically, and emotionally) can help with relaxation, milk production, positional comfort, neck/back tension, and can decrease body/breast tenderness to name a few of the common benefits.

For baby, it can improve latch and suckling, eliminate discrepancy in latch from breast to breast, calm an over-stimulated nervous system, reduce reflux, and soothe colic amongst other benefits.

In truth, rather than treating a list of specific conditions or symptoms, chiropractic aims to restore balance and ease to the body so it can do exactly what it was meant to do naturally—thrive.

Dr. Bari's message for mothers experiencing breastfeeding grief

Breastfeeding is a primal, natural, seemingly intuitive act, but it is also a dance that needs to be learned by both mama and baby. Some pairs seem to gravitate very naturally into the steps and rhythms. For others, it takes guidance, practice, and patience. Neither situation indicates a greater or lesser level of love or innate ability to parent—it is simply part of your unique story together.

Sometimes, despite a mom's and baby's best efforts, breastfeeding isn't possible and this can be very hard on the heart. Wherever you are on your journey together, know that you are not alone and that support comes in many forms. It goes without saying that moms who receive support from partners, family members, other women, and/or practitioners have an easier time learning and navigating this dance. Never be afraid or ashamed to ask for the help you need.

If you are interested in working with a chiropractor near you who is committed to pregnancy and pediatric care, go to: www.icpa4kids.org

Click on the "Find A Chiropractor" link.

JoAnn Lewis, Infant Massage – The Power is in our Hands

LMT, CEIM, Director & Educator of the Family Massage Education Center in Ashland, Oregon

www.hellofmec.com

JoAnn Lewis is a mother and grandmother. She has a teaching degree, is a licensed massage therapist, a certified educator of infant massage for parents and their babies, and an IAIM Trainer of infant massage instructors. She is also the owner and director of the Family Massage Education Center in Ashland, Oregon.

Hilary: You are the go-to person for infant massage here in the Rogue Valley. I've heard that you have a personal story about that?

JoAnn: Yes, I do. I had a little boy who was an emergency cesarean birth, and he was very colicky. We tried everything, from gripe waters to medicines, driving around, walking around. But whatever we tried, it would soothe him for ten minutes at most and then he was crying again. When a midwife showed me the stomach strokes of infant massage, he began to improve! Day by day, as he got better and better, I felt incredible relief. I wondered: Why hadn't the doctor shown me this? Why didn't everybody know this?

I wanted to know more, so I went to massage school, received training from the International Association of Infant Massage program, and became a trainer with that same association. Today, we have sixty trainers teaching in over fifty countries!

This is what I learned: as a culture, we have forgotten how to touch with true permission and respect. There is a lot of fear regarding touch. Many of us actually crave to experience what respectful touching looks and feels like. Optimally, everyone could benefit in knowing how to speak the language of touch. We can do so much for each other through the power that is in our hands, directly, without fear, without holding back, but also with respect, with permission.

This is why I opened the Family Massage Education Center. We're teaching parent and baby classes, pregnant partner classes, couples classes, and singles classes – ongoing, every day of the week.

Hilary: Do you have other examples of benefits for babies?

JoAnn: My best example is a family who took the training with their last two of seven children. The father had been away for two tours in Afghanistan. He had missed a lot, and he needed that bonding.

Five years later, the mother told me, "You know, JoAnn, my two younger children are just different people. At first, I thought it was because they were the youngest. But then I realized, they are the first to adapt to any situation. They are the first ones to come and help. They are the first to ask permission. They are sensitive and can read the cues of other people, just like we do in infant massage. And I know why. It's because of the infant massage."

Hilary: Are you saying that when babies experience respectful touch themselves, that this respectful behavior becomes part of their personality?

Oh yes. The baby's nervous system learns by absorbing the patterns of the caregivers. If the baby's earliest experience includes daily sessions of respectful, communicative touching, think what that means!

We know that when people are more connected, as parents and children during massage, we are better adjusted, psychologically, emotionally, and physically. Add to that the benefits of right-left brain integration with massage, (touch and movement that crosses over the midline of the body, so that the brain is activated to integrate its left and right sides), and you'll see a beautiful development of personality and a more stable individual.

When you start looking at the scientific research, it's amazing. Take this example: Babies who are born prematurely have 49% more weight gain per day just by getting physical touch from their parents, 10-15 minutes, 2 -3 times a day. They go home in half the time. It's a huge dollar saving to parents and hospitals. And think, what if we took that idea and transferred it to the so-called "normal" family? Wouldn't they be going to the emergency room less often? Wouldn't they be healthier, smarter, and happier people?

Hilary: JoAnn, if you could speak directly to the readers of my book, what would you like to say?

JoAnn: Keep touching! Touch is the first language, and massage is the extension of that.

Think about the film *Babies*. It followed the first year of four babies from different parts of the world. While the film doesn't show it directly, clearly, the babies from Africa and Mongolia have received infant massage. You don't get such exquisite muscle tone from genetics alone, or the ability to balance a cup on your head as you begin walking. That's normally the result of lots of stimulation and right-left brain integration through infant massage.

And if a mother is breastfeeding, massage activates the baby's food absorption hormones to be able to absorb that food well, absorb all the nutrients out of it, to build a stronger body.

And just think if we massage babies who, for whatever reason, are not breastfed. It would be so much better. Because there are circumstances beyond choice, beyond control, where babies are bottle fed, but we still have the power in our hands to communicate, bond, and support our child's overall development, health and immunity with our loving, respectful touch.

Also, I would like to say that a lot of people have problems touching and bonding if they've not had it themselves in their own past, or if they were neglected or abused. . . and infant massage, and massage for anyone, can be a chance to heal those kinds of scars.

We actually teach infant massage at most of the military bases now. It turns out that the highest rate of suicide in the military is for returnees who miss the birth of a child. The purpose of infant massage at the military base is to get that skin-on-skin bonding time, that closeness, that communication going from the very beginning when the father returns. They teach baby carrying techniques to get the dads doing skin-on-skin, wearing their babies, and doing the baby massage right away. Now, Dad is part of the family again. He is back in the fold. Remember to keep touching with love, permission and respect! Let's make a better world for the next generation with massage for everyone.

DR. BOBBY GHAHERI, PASSIONATE SURGEON WITH INSIGHT

Dr. Bob Ghaheri is a board certified ENT surgeon with a clinical focus on breastfeeding medicine.

Hilary: Did you have a personal experience that motivated you to specialize in breastfeeding medicine?

Dr. Bob Ghaheri: Yes, my first daughter had severe problems breastfeeding. We visited numerous lactation consultants and our pediatrician, and never received an answer. Despite this, my very determined wife nursed my daughter for years.

We then had another daughter, this time at home. Our midwives suspected a problem when the same severe pain developed for my wife. We worked with a lactation consultant who noticed the correlation with my daughter's tongue-tie. We had it clipped at day seven, and immediately things changed.

I became upset that this wasn't part of my education as an ENT surgeon, and that the LC's we'd seen the first time around hadn't seen the tongue-tie. And so I dove in.

Hilary: How would you describe your work with breastfeeding infants?

Dr. Bobby Ghaheri: I see babies in the office who have difficulty with their latch from tongue-tie and lip-tie. I perform laser-assisted tongue-tie and lip-tie releases to allow the babies a better chance at a successful latch.

Basically, my procedures allow the vast majority of babies who are unable to latch the chance to latch on. Otherwise, they wean.

Hilary: Speaking directly to the readers of my book, what would you like to say?

Dr. Bobby Ghaheri: The main message I would send to moms is that if you feel that something isn't right with your experience with breastfeeding, start searching. Your doctor has hundreds of other patients to care for. Same goes for your LC. So the most invested person in your breastfeeding relationship is you. There is nothing more significant in a child's well being than breastfeeding, so everything should be done to maintain. If your doctor/LC is dismissing your concerns, then it's reasonable to switch providers to find someone who will support you.

LISA MARASCO, SUPPORT FOR COMPLEX ISSUES

Lisa Marasco has an MA in Human Development with specialization in Lactation Consulting. She is an IBCLC, and a fellow of the professional organization ILCA. She is a co-author of the book *A Breastfeeding Mother's Guide to Making More Milk.*

Lisa is known for her energy and advocacy for research and education regarding solutions to breastfeeding issues such as tongue-tie, insufficient glandular tissue and true low milk supply.

Hilary: What in your personal life motivated you to work in this field?

Lisa: My own children! I fell in love with breastfeeding and what it taught me about motherhood, but was dismayed to see struggling friends throwing in the towel. I first became a La Leche Leader in order to help, and then discovered that I had a passion for the clinical side of lactation problems and made the decision to become a consultant. I just wanted other mothers to experience the wonders of breastfeeding as I did.

Hilary: How do you see and support mothers going through breastfeeding grief in your practice?

Lisa: I validate their pain and their right to grieve. So many mothers are told to buck up and move on and just be grateful that they have a healthy baby. Few people acknowledge the death of a mother's dream of how life with baby would go, and especially about having a trouble-free breastfeeding relationship. Some mothers feel judged by family and friends, who seem to suggest that they just need to try a little harder. So I tell them that their feelings are valid, that they can tell these people that the lactation consultant says the mother is doing everything possible, and I suggest limiting contact with naysayers for a while.

Hilary: What would you like to say to the reader of this book?

Lisa: You have a right to grieve. We live in an imperfect world and this is not how breastfeeding is supposed to go. Do what you are able to do, and make peace with the situation.

BEVERLY MORGAN IBCLC, HEALING HER INNER CHILD, HELPING MOTHERS AND BABIES

Beverly: I am an Internationally Board Certified Lactation Consultant. I have been in the breastfeeding field since 1973, first as a breastfeeding mother, then as a La Leche League Leader. I sat for the IBCLC exam the second year it was offered and have continually worked in the field since that time.

Hilary: What motivated you to become a lactation consultant?

Beverly: Shortly after I was married, I met a woman who was breastfeeding her baby. As she talked to me about breastfeeding it seemed like a good choice. I had not even considered it. I did not know anyone who had breastfed a baby and I knew lots of families with babies.

She told me that La Leche League was a good place to go for breastfeeding help. I attended a meeting before my daughter was born and gained confidence, as I saw many women breastfeeding their children. As my baby grew, I came to realize that breastfeeding is about much more than food; it is part of a very powerful relationship between mother and child.

As a motherless child, whose mother died giving birth to me, I know how important a mother is in a child's life. It is not true that you don't miss what you do not have. There are examples around you to constantly remind you of what you have missed. As many who experience grief know, helping others can be part of your own healing. Helping mothers and babies to have that breast-nurturing bond continues to be healing for me.

Hilary: What are your experiences helping mothers who are going through breastfeeding grief?

Beverly: When mothers do not achieve their deeply cherished dream of breastfeeding their baby, they often feel they have let down their baby. They are saddened and feel betrayed by their body, and by a society that assumes anyone can easily feed a baby, after all, "it is natural"

Sometimes, mothers who have a successful breastfeeding relationship assume that the unsuccessful mother just did not try hard enough, or that she secretly did not value breastfeeding, or that she was too lazy or did not really want the best for her baby. Mothers who are bottle-feeding formula may also feel that the mother who tries to breastfeed is somehow looking down on her choice to use formula. She is seen as part of the enemy camp. This leaves the grieving mother without a support community.

In 1999, I and one of the mothers who was living in the no-man's land of formula feeding and grieving for her breastfeeding relationship began an online support group called Mothers Overcoming Breastfeeding Issues (MOBI). The group was started as a grief group for those who had not met their breastfeeding goals. The mothers were surprised and comforted to find other mothers who had similar experiences. Their grief was easier to handle when they were not alone, and their mutual support enabled some mothers to find solutions and to turn their breastfeeding relationship around.

Hilary: What would you like to say to the mothers who are reading this book?

Beverly: My wish is that every mother meets her breastfeeding goals and that every baby can experience the joys and comfort of breast-nurturing at mom's breasts. I would urge every mother to tirelessly search for answers as to what is causing the difficulties and to take comfort in what she and her baby have achieved together. Be sure to look for an IBCLC, as we have the rigorous education and certification that is needed to assess complex situations.

Sometimes, a mother cannot provide all the milk the baby needs, or the baby cannot manage to get the milk he needs at her breasts, or mom might be on a medication that does not allow her to breastfeed. These situations bring anguish and mothers need a safe place to work through the grief.

Grief needs to be gone through, it cannot be avoided. However, there are many years of parenthood ahead. As the years go by, the storms of grief in the baby days seem to be more of a passing storm, and the good memories do get sweeter.

I would like to say that a baby needs mom and loves mom, and does not judge her as harshly as she judges herself. Fashion your breastfeeding relationship in a way that it brings you comfort. Babies nurse for relationship and food, and even if there is not a full supply or a baby cannot drain the breasts effectively, a baby may still breastfeed for comfort.

Wise MOBI moms say: Don't quit on your worst day. You may regret it later. On a day that is not so hard, if you still think it is time to quit, you will be less likely to have long-term bitter regrets. You will then be more able to focus on how hard you tried, and to treasure the shining moments when breastfeeding seemed to be working, and you can look forward to the many adventures ahead. I wish you all the happy parenting and the wonderful memories our children give us.

ANNA HUMPHREYS, PRENATAL MEDITATION FOR ENERGETIC COMMUNICATION WITH BABY

Doula, Infant massage teacher, Calm Birth Instructor (Prenatal Meditation)

www.southernoregonbirthconnections.com/doulas

Anna Humphreys is a doula (CD DONA), an infant massage teacher, and an instructor in Calm Birth—a form of prenatal meditation that is based on Tibetan Buddhism, and that develops both mindfulness and an energetic connection between a mother and her child. Calm Birth features two CDs, Calm Birth and Calm Mothering, and also a book, Calm Birth: New Method for Conscious Childbirth, all of which can be purchased online.

Currently, Anna is completing her BS in psychology and preparing for postgraduate studies. She plans to explore how prenatal experiences affect infants, and to study the impact of prenatal meditation on the baby and parents as well as its possible value for society as a whole.

Anna teaches Calm Birth to mothers in her community, and reaches mothers around the world through Skype.

Hilary: What motivates you to do this work?

Anna: I am a "meditator baby." My parents met at a meditation retreat, and my mother meditated twice a day during her pregnancy with me. When I began to meditate at age nineteen, it immediately changed me—turned my world around! I recognized that I had been hardwired for meditation in the womb, and that I love it.

I sincerely feel that as a meditator baby, I am blessed to have come into this earth without too much pre-existing trauma. I want to share these blessings through my work with families, and also through research.

Hilary: What makes Calm Birth different from other forms of meditation or mindfulness practices?

Anna: Calm Birth teaches many components of mindfulness that are known to reduce stress and stop the fight-or-flight response, but Calm Birth is unique in that it has been developed especially for mothers. For instance, the relaxation part takes you deep into the anatomy of your entire body including your womb, and it puts you in touch with your baby's presence. Then, there is a strong emphasis on breathing into the energy center in your abdomen, breathing into your womb, connecting with your baby with your breath, and sending your baby energy with your breath, and bonding that way.

Hilary: Have you seen concrete benefits for your clients?

Anna: My meditation students sometimes ask me to act as their doula, so I can see the benefits of Calm Birth first-hand.

Many of the moms who are attracted to Calm Birth had a traumatic first birth, with postpartum depression and breastfeeding problems, and they want to feel empowered this time. These mothers often say that they felt held in their power center during this birth experience and were able to respond to whatever came up during the birth process.

Just recently, one mother told me that as long as she stuck with the breathing, she did not feel any pain. She felt sensation, but not pain. If she was distracted from her breathing focus she felt pain that could be overwhelming, but she could transition out of the pain when she focused on her breath again. By being able to return to her center, and to her breathing, she said she was able to have the birth of her dreams.

Another mother had had four previous natural births, but she needed an emergency cesarean birth or her fifth. Afterwards, she was separated from her baby for three hours. Yet, she still tells me that this was the best birth she had had. She says that because she meditated throughout the pregnancy, and during the emergency situation was able to stay in her center, and stay with her baby, and breathe energy to her baby, she thinks that Calm Birth helped them establish a deep bond.

It's also good for mothers to know that if they have a cesarean birth, their immune system has been strengthened by meditation, and they will have more resistance to bacteria in the hospital.

And then there are also many first-time mammas who, whether their birth was smooth or challenging, tell me how wonderful it was to have bonded with their child during pregnancy, because they felt very close with their baby after the birth.

Hilary: What does Calm Birth offer mothers who are experiencing breastfeeding grief?

Anna: There's the nutritional aspect of breastfeeding, and the closeness, but for people who can't have that, for whatever reason, it's empowering to know that there are still ways you can be physically and energetically close to your baby.

Hilary: Which is what I emphasize in this book.

Anna: Exactly! That's why I think you work is important, because it is not just seeing breastfeeding and bonding one right way. It's about acknowledging the grief that comes with these challenges, but ultimately discovering how those challenges can bring us closer with our children, and ourselves.

Hilary: Could a mother come to you after birth and learn the meditation practices that are helpful after birth, called Calm Mothering?

Anna: Absolutely, it's never too late. Whether your child is two weeks old or twenty, you can learn these practices, enhance your own sense of self, and bond with your child energetically. If a woman is having breastfeeding issues, the Calm Mother breastfeeding practice can be really empowering. Just relaxing your body can help your milk flow. And if that doesn't happen, you can still "breath-feed" your baby.

The Calm Mothering breastfeeding practice that I teach is called "Breast-Breathing, Breath-Feeding," and it's perfect for nourishing yourself and your baby from your heart and from your deep energy center.

Hilary: If you could speak now to mothers who are suffering, if you could reach out and talk to them, what would you like to say?

Anna: The words that come to mind are just be gentle. Be gentle with yourself; be gentle with your child.

Cheryl Scott, Hospital Lactation Consultant with Heart

RN, PhD, IBCLC

www.cherylscottspeakerservices.weekbly.com

I have been a hospital-based IBCLC for thirty years at Kaiser in Oakland and Sacramento. I am a national lecturer and teacher of new methods of breastfeeding support and interventions at ILCA and PESI conferences. I am honored to contribute to this much-needed book by Hilary Jacobson.

Heart to Heart Time with Mom and Dad

Mothers and fathers often feel sad or distraught when birth or breastfeeding do not go as planned. It is good to know that through heart to heart contact, parents and babies can forge the desired bond and heal their hurt emotions, simply from snuggling their baby close to their heart.

Science affirms the powerful effect of heart to heart contact. The benefits include: two hours less crying per 24 hours; longer sleep in-between feedings if mom or dad holds their baby for about 20 minutes before placing their baby down to sleep (this is long enough for baby to get into a good REM level of sleep), and a reduction of the risk of SIDS.

Studies encourage both fathers and mothers to hold their baby close to their heart for at least 4 hours each day for the first 6-8 weeks after childbirth. It's easy for breastfeeding mothers to achieve 4 hours each day because usually the baby's heart is directly across from mother's heart when the baby is held in the cradle hold. And if the mother burps her child after each feeding, she is usually holding her baby over her heart in a semi-upright position as well. Mothers who supplement using a bottle can hold their baby close to their heart and have gentle, loving eye contact with their baby. At other times, mothers can hold their baby on their chest, heart to heart, with as much direct skin on skin as often as possible to allow for deep bonding.

Heart to heart contact with the father is also very important. If the mother is recovering from birth or is fatigued, a father can be a great source of comfort to her and his baby—and also give comfort to himself—by the practice of heart to heart connection.

From the website, kangaroocare.com:

Benefits of skin-to-skin contact for Dads!

o   You will be empowered to care for your baby and not feel helpless or useless or redundant.

o   You will become central to the caring team

o   Better bonding

o   Emotional healing

o   You are calmer

o   Able to read your baby's unique cues for hunger or stress

o   You can get more sleep

Holding your baby close to your heart produces high levels of oxytocin, a hormone that reduces stress and anxiety in mother, father and baby, and that promotes feelings of happiness and wellness. This hormone allows mother, father and baby to fall quickly into a deep sleep, which scientists say is equal to a full night's sleep—even if it is only a 2-hour nap.

I am so happy whenever I talk to parents about heart to heart contact. I have found that even those mothers who are not able to successfully breastfeed establish deep bonding and feelings of enhanced love and joy with their newborn baby by cuddling heart to heart many hours each day.
–Cheryl Scott RN, PhD, IBCLC

VALERIE BANARIE, HYPNOTHERAPY FOR MOTHERS ENDURING SEPARATION FROM THEIR BABIES

RN, BA in Social Work and Sociology, Lactation Consultant in Private Practice, Certified in Clinical Hypnotherapy

In the twenty-five years I have been a lactation consultant working with new mothers and their babies, I have helped countless women deal with the grief and despair that occurs when their baby (or babies) need to be in the NICU (neonatal intensive care unit), and when their babies sometimes cannot go home with them when the mothers are discharged.

Babies are separated from their mothers and placed in the NICU for many reasons. Some babies are in the NICU because of specific medical issues that need to be addressed in an intensive way, and others are there for observation if a problem is suspected, or if they are very small or prematurely born babies, which is especially common with twins or triplets. Premature babies often lack the strength needed to stay awake and suckle at the breast or bottle, and so they must receive nourishment by feeding tube.

It is heartbreaking to see your baby in the NICU, and, in some cases, depending upon the reason they are there, to not be able to hold or touch your newborn. Almost every new mother and father in this situation feels helpless and distanced from their baby. This can be demoralizing, and parents often fear that they will never be able to mother their baby the way they so desperately want to.

Often, mothers feel overwhelming guilt and self-anger that they might have caused the situation by something that they did or did not do during pregnancy. These emotions are very real and very troubling.

Being able to enjoy skin-on-skin with their baby, called "kangaroo care," helps relieve the parent's pain and brings connection with their baby. Some mothers and fathers may also need extra help, such as counseling or other therapy to help them move through the feelings of helplessness, sadness and guilt.

It is a truly difficult situation. More new parents than I can count have told me that they feel like their baby is not theirs, but belongs to the NICU staff. It is easy to understand how such feelings can occur, when someone else does everything for your baby as you sit on the sidelines and watch. As your baby grows stronger and starts to overcome whatever challenges there have been, you will be shown how to care for him or her yourself, and allowed to spend time in kangaroo care, providing skin-to-skin with your baby.

Many mothers experience difficulties providing breastmilk for their babies in NICU, and this is easy to understand. The feelings of separation, worry, and guilt, plus the hospital environment, are not exactly conducive to milk flow. Be sure to have an appointment with your hospital lactation consultant, and be sure that the pump is a good fit. Some mothers also use a medication called Domperidone, or special milk-enhancing herbs, and/or lactogenic foods to support their supply.

If mothers are not able to produce milk at this time, it may still be possible to re-lactate and restore the breastfeeding relationship, fully or partially, later on. In the meantime, skin-on-skin and heart-to-heart connection will give you and your baby the bonding and loving time you need, and this is also supportive of your baby's emotions, brain and immune system.

As a hypnotherapist, I know the value of visualization to help the emotions heal. The visualization that I provide below is useful for mothers who are pumping in NICU, to help them produce milk in the hospital environment, and for mothers who are healing from separation from their babies.

A Visualization for Deep Connection

Sit or lay comfortably somewhere you are unlikely to be disturbed for a little while.

Close your eyes and become aware of your breathing. Observe as you gently breathe in and out. Breathe as if you are filling your belly with air every time you inhale, allowing your deep breath to start there and expand to fill your lungs. Everyone has a rate and rhythm of breathing that allows for maximum relaxation and finding yours is easy. Experiment until you find the one that works best for you.

Once you are breathing deeply, slowly and comfortably, imagine that, streaming from the ceiling to the top of your head is a warm, relaxing, loving light that relaxes everything that it touches. Imagine what it would be like for this light to allow your scalp at the top of your head to relax and let go of any stress or tension. Everyone imagines differently, so you may see the light or simply get an impression that it is there. However you experience this is exactly correct for you at this time.

Imagine what it would be like for this light to move down your face, over your eyelids, relaxing every tiny muscle that surrounds your eyes. You may notice your eyelids twitching a bit. This is one indication of relaxation, and in a few moments you will be unaware of it, even as your eyelids and face continue to relax deeper and deeper.

Imagine what it would be like for this wonderful light to shine upon the joint that connects your upper and lower jaws, that place where we might tend to store so much tension. Imagine the muscles being bathed in warm relaxing light and allow those muscles to relax. Perhaps they will relax so much that your mouth might open slightly in the next few minutes.

Imagine this light moving to your shoulders, massaging them with warmth. Allow yourself to sink even more comfortably into what you are resting upon as the light moves down from your shoulders to your elbows, from your elbows to your wrists. . . and from your wrists to the tips of each and every finger.

Bring your attention to the nape of your neck, the top of your spine and imagine what it would be like for this wonderful light to move down your spine in a column of light, all the way down to your waist. Now imagine this light spreading from your spine all around your torso, relaxing all the muscles between each and every rib. Notice that as those muscles relax, your breathing becomes even more perfect in its ability to relax you deeper and deeper with every breath, as easily, effortlessly and naturally as breathing itself.

Now imagine this light traveling from your waist to your knees, and from your knees to your ankles. . . and now from your ankles to the tips of each and every toe.

Take a moment and give yourself permission to allow yourself this opportunity to release anything that is less than completely comfortable and relaxing. The more comfortable you are, the deeper you relax, and the deeper you relax the more comfortable you become.

Take a very deep, slow breath and as you inhale allow the light to travel to and envelop any part of you that might need a bit more relaxing. As you exhale, release anything that no longer serves you. Repeat this two more times.

Continuing to breathe at your perfect rate and rhythm, imagine yourself surrounded by a bubble of warm light. From top to bottom, from side to side. Imagine yourself so comfortably within this wonderful bubble. Perhaps the bubble is a specific color. Perhaps it is white, or perhaps you only have a vague understanding that it is there. However you experience it is exactly correct for you. If you wish, enclose the other parent or someone of your choosing inside the bubble with you.

Inside this bubble is peace and comfort. Think of your baby now. If you have an article of your baby's clothing with you, inhale your baby's beautiful scent and let it fill you as you inhale deeply. Let yourself feel your love for your baby, and let your love fill the bubble completely. Take a few moments to enjoy being wrapped securely in this love.

Now imagine that with you still inside it, the bubble is expanding to include your baby within it. It is completely unimportant how physically distant you may be from the baby.

Just allow the bubble to surround you and the image of your baby that you hold in your mind. Breathe in the scent of your baby, and imagine holding your baby in your arms and smelling the sweet smell of your baby's head. Feel the downy soft hair as it brushes against your lips and allow the love you feel for your baby to fill the bubble even more fully. You and your baby are bonded by this love. Feel the love your baby has for you as well. Your bubble is full of love you share and the amount is limitless.

You can imagine a light flowing from your heart to your baby's heart with you both inside the bubble. If there is another person with you, imagine the light connecting to them as well. Allow this light to bind you even more securely to each other, and this connection grows stronger each time you do this.

Take as much time to enjoy this love and connection as you wish. When you are ready, slowly count to three and open your eyes, feeling and knowing that you and your baby are connected deeply and infinitely by love. Regardless of physical distance, you are together always.

© Valerie Banarie, 2014

COELI DWIVEDI, CONSTELLATION WORK FOR THE FAMILY

www.familyconstellation.works

www.coelidwivedi.com

www.integratingwellness.net

Coeli Dwivedi is a wellness coach and health educator with a background in midwifery, somatic healing and family constellation work. She has four children, all born at home, and was a homebirth midwife for twenty years. She has recently completed her MS in health education, and currently works with women and families in the postpartum, or one to two years after childbirth.

Hilary: What motivated you to become a midwife?

Coeli: I had such an empowering and safe birth experience with a midwife, and as part of that experience, I felt a nagging sense that more women need to be able to have access to this type of birth.

Today, I primarily work with women in the postpartum period, helping mothers transition into motherhood with confidence and trust in themselves and their inner knowing.

Hilary: How do you support women through breastfeeding grief?

Coeli: I look at the whole woman, at her diet, sleep patterns, stress level, her fears, if she's getting any exercise, her feelings about being a mother, sharing her body all the time with he baby. . . I set her up with resources as needed, and also target what she needs that I can support.

For instance, maybe her stress is that she doesn't have money for food, and I will connect her into those resources that are there to help. Maybe she is depressed, or she feels overwhelmed, or unsure of herself, and I will help her develop confidence in her abilities. In the great majority of the women I've served, breastfeeding problems are also a confidence issue.

Then, I do a basic assessment on baby's wellness, which includes the latch, tongue-tie, and if the baby is getting milk. If anything is outside of normal or is questionable, I refer the mother to an IBCLC lactation consultant. I love having a team of people to work with.

Beyond that, even if breastfeeding is going well, some mothers experience deep grief that goes unaddressed, and that stands in the way of experiencing the joy and receiving the gift of mothering. I have found that somatic healing processes, including bioenergetics and family constellation work, can be profoundly healing for this.

Hilary: Do you offer your work online, via Skype or other system?

Coeli: Yes, and I'm happy to say that it's still powerful work, whether phone or Skype. If you're local, I prefer face-to-face interaction. However, I understand that it's sometimes hard for moms to leave the house, and so I'm open to do phone or Skype with local mothers as well. I also travel to do group constellation work for a family.

Hilary: What would you like to say to the reader of this book?

Coeli: I just want to encourage you, that if you're grieving or feeling depressed, and even if you can't quite put your finger on what you're feeling or why, reach out. There are lots of people who can help you, people who not only have the tools and training to help you, but who are devoting their lives to supporting women and families at this time.

If you would like to learn more about how family constellation work can help you, please contact me through my website.

CHANTI JOY SMITH, BIRTH TRAUMA RESOLUTION, BREASTFEEDING HEALING AND SUPPORT

CPM, SEP, www.embodiedbeginnings.com

Chanti Joy Smith is a homebirth midwife, Somatic Experiencing Practitioner, Pre and Perinatal Birth Therapist (Castellino Method), a bodyworker of twenty years specializing in craniosacral therapy and Body-Mind Centering (Bonnie Bainbridge Cohen), a lactation specialist, western trained herbalist and flower essence practitioner.

Hilary: What drew you to this field with mothers and babies, what motivates you?

Chantia: First, I would like to express my deep gratitude for all of my teachers, colleagues, students and families who have taught me how to support moms and babies. My mom and stepfather are therapists, and my father was a human rights activist. I was raised surrounded by a sense of compassion and service, and I've always wanted to make a difference in the world. As a midwife, I wanted to be sure I wasn't bringing any of my own unresolved issues into the birth room, and I looked into ways to do my own deep healing. In healing my birth wounds, I learned how to better support others in their healing. I am a lifelong learner, a dedicated teacher, and I am committed to offering the best support I can to my clients.

Hilary: Have you seen many mothers with breastfeeding challenges?

Chantia: Yes. I work mostly with mothers postpartum to integrate their births, help them heal any trauma, and resolve difficult lactation issues. It's not uncommon for parents to be referred to me by a lactation consultant, midwife or doula, and usually, after our session, the baby can latch. I also work with babies before and after tongue-tie release, to support the functionality of their suck and swallow reflex and help maintain the new pattern.

Hilary: Can you explain more about how you work with clients?

Chanti: Often I find that the problem is related to an interruption in the sequencing of birth events—a time or situation in the birth process where the baby got stuck, or where drugs were used, or where the baby's natural introduction to the breast was stalled or prevented, so that the baby was unable to latch with ease in the natural sequence.

Craniosacral therapy or bodywork can help unwind and release tension in a baby's body. They might also need to be guided—with cranial touch— through what we call the "process of supported attachment," or the "breast crawl," which is the way babies attach when left to their own instincts after birth. While re-enacting this "journey," a baby can tell the story of its birth, showing the birth movements with its body, and integrating any of the hard places of the birth experience. This allows the baby to re-pattern its responses for the natural initiation of breastfeeding. With its tension resolved, the baby can nurse with a good latch and more ease.

I help mothers, too. This is important, because mothers and babies are deeply connected. In Pre and Perinatal Birth Therapy we say, "If mom settles, baby settles." Often, a mother may be feeling a lot of grief or trauma from the birth or her breastfeeding challenges. She's probably been told, "You have a healthy baby. You're healthy. You should be happy." Yet, she's holding inside herself this deep despair that things hadn't worked out the way she envisioned. Maybe she's also holding tension in her body because of some procedure she had to go through. In order to be fully present for herself and her baby, mothers need to be able to feel those feelings and release them in a safe and supported way.

Hilary: With your wide range of tools, is there a special technique that you often use with breastfeeding grief?

Chanti: Yes, I often do somatic work with mothers. Somatic work brings awareness to sensations in the body. It looks at how we hold tension or trauma in the actual tissues in our body, as well as orienting us to our inherent health. Through this work, tension can be released and mothers can deeply relax and settle.

Also, we might explore any generational trauma as well as the health in the ancestral lineage—becoming aware of epigenetic influences through the family line. As we get in touch with the body's innate intelligence, and with the trust and the health that are held in the body's cellular knowing, mothers naturally shift from a state of anxiety to one of being settled. To help with healing generational trauma around breastfeeding I might begin by asking, "How far back do we have to go to find someone in your lineage who was breastfed so we can find and feel, in that cellular memory, that healthy breastfeeding relationship?"

Many mothers find that after deep somatic remembering and working with supported attachment, their challenges resolve. And if a mother wasn't breastfed herself, she now has an opportunity to give her baby a gift that is different than what she had.

Hilary: Do you work with mothers on Skype?

Chanti: If women can't find someone in their community to do a home visit, I will meet them on Skype and support them, identifying and releasing trauma, leading them through re-patterning of the birth and breastfeeding sequences, perhaps doing somatic therapy, whatever is needed.

Hilary: What would you like to say to the reader of this book?

Chanti: I get it. You've been working too hard, and too long, and you just want to be able to feed your baby. This is the most primal instinct, to give nourishment to life that you have created, and it's painful to not be able to do that, or to be struggling as much as you have been.

I wish that I could take you into a room full of mothers and have them hold you in your grief, because you are not alone. There are many who feel like you, yet there are also many who have moved through and beyond this struggle, and I would love to have you sit with them, as well.

There was a mom, who couldn't breastfeed for four months, and then, with persistence, her little one latched on. So it can happen. Whatever happens for you, however you decide to be, as a mother, providing nourishment for your baby, what is most important is that you make sense of it for yourself, that you find peace, stay connected to your little one and know you did the best you could.

Jennifer Tow, IBCLC, RLC, Difficult Cases

Holistic IBCLC, holisticibclc.blogspot.com

Jennifer, an IBCLC of 25 years, has pioneered protocols that address the structural, nutritional, digestive and epigenetic issues behind breastfeeding problems. Her clients frequently suffer from chronic health problems, intestinal problems, autoimmune disorders, and struggle with methylation and other epigenetic stressors. Her philosophy is: "Heal the Mother, Heal the Baby." Jennifer provides one-on-one support, and she provides education and training through online webinars, for parents and professionals.

Hilary: Hi Jennifer, did you have a personal experience of breastfeeding grief?

Jennifer: Yes. . . I sure did! Ok, a bit of background. . . I was fortunate in that my sister had breastfed her son, and so, even though no one else in our family had nursed, I had a sense that it was normal. When I began to nurse and to understand more about what it does for the mother and baby, I asked my mother about her breastfeeding choices. . . and she told me that she had never even considered it. Her story was that her older brother had been very ill as a baby, and that her mother was told it was because of breastfeeding. Her mother hadn't nursed her subsequent children, including my mother, and so for my mother, breastfeeding was not even given a second thought.

I remember one day, I was sitting on the couch, nursing my son who was six weeks old, and I started to cry. I couldn't stop the tears. I am tearing up now just talking about it. . . I just cried and cried and all the time I was thinking, "My mother will never experience this. And I never experienced this with my mother."

At the time I was overcoming a lot of stuff from my childhood, and it came to me that I didn't know how I would have found a path into motherhood without breastfeeding. It was that big.

Suddenly, I had a lot of compassion for my mother. I felt her loss, our loss. And even now, I tear up.

It hit me like a truck. I was a new mother, six weeks postpartum. I was not a lactation consultant of 25 years with all my knowledge about the value of breastfeeding. But that's how it hit me—like a truck. I couldn't stop the tears.

And yet, talking about it now, I find myself holding back a little bit about how powerful that is for me. In our society, people aren't supposed to talk about how powerful breastfeeding is because that supposedly means we are challenging or diminishing someone else's experience or choice. But how can one person's experience challenge that of another? And how is it helpful to not have a right to your emotions?

Hilary: "We can't heal what we can't feel."

Jennifer: Yes! And also, our society wants me to say that it doesn't make that much difference if I was breastfed or not, because so many people, also people in the medical community, are unable or unwilling to acknowledge the depth of motherhood.

That is why I do what I do. Because I can't imagine having lived my life and having mothered my children without that . . . (pause) . . . experience. But no, it's more than an "experience." It's not like an afternoon in the park. (Pause.) Here's what it is: I can't imagine not having had that life. It just—, it weaves you. Every time you nurse that baby, fabric is woven. You become through it.

And I can really understand why this wound of breastfeeding grief is difficult to move past for so many mothers—because it is a wound that is left gaping, not allowed to be addressed. Because we hear, "What do you mean, that's a wound! You shouldn't feel bad about that!"

I think of the herbalist Jeannine Parvati Baker, who said that all of a mother's love, and all of a mother's tears, get mixed together and made into her milk. It's true. And in this sense, too, breastmilk and breastfeeding is humanizing, because all of you goes into it. So if you are feeling that wound, it takes a lot of courage, to bleed while you nurse, in a sense.

Hilary: And by bleed you mean, to be fully present with your pain—and your joy.

Jennifer: That's it.

Hilary: Jennifer, I have heard that your private practice today focuses mostly on difficult-to-solve breastfeeding situations. Is that true?

Jennifer: Yes, though it wasn't always like that. I began as a La Leche League leader, doing what I love most: peer-to-peer support. But because I am a careful observer, I soon came to appreciate the complexity that underlies many breastfeeding challenges. Today, mothers with especially complex problems seek me out. Often, these mothers' crises have been building for a long time. They've not been sitting around, casually waiting for the volcano to erupt—they have been actively seeking to avert disaster, they have been looking for help. But beyond receiving emotional support, they haven't found the information they need.

Some of these kids are really in bad shape. I mean serious weeping eczema, failure to thrive, screaming for hours on end, day after day. And often when they find me the mothers say, "I'm at a crossroads. My gastroenterologist/pediatrician/allergist wants me to wean my baby to elemental formula. And it's breaking my heart."

What they are asking is if there is any way I can validate that their breastmilk isn't harming their baby. It's truly heartbreaking.

And the first thing that I say is "Don't stop breastfeeding." I want them to receive this message: formula may remove something that is irritating to your baby, for sure. But it doesn't give your baby the stem-cells, the antibodies, growth factors, hormones, flora, all these amazing components—and you won't be giving the breastfeeding relationship. And I tell them that this is not a worthy tradeoff.

We can fix the components that irritate the baby by addressing the mother's and baby's gut health. We can look at structural problems. Tongue-tie, it turns out, is often at the surface of something much deeper, having to do with more global "airway" problems. A lot of these infants are mouth breathing, they are snoring, and they have a dysregulated autonomic nervous system, which of course affects their feeding patterns and their digestion.

Hilary: So you fix the structural problems and all of a sudden the baby no longer has colic, their latch and suck patterns are right, and they can build the mom's milk supply?

Jennifer: That's right. But not enough doctors or lactation consultants are looking at the larger picture. The focus for them is on feeding. But before feeding, the organism needs to breathe. And if we don't address these problems, that baby is at risk to have sleeping problems, cognitive and behavior problems, and learning disorders. It's huge—and there's so much we can do to help.

Hilary: What would you like to see happen in our society as a result of your work, and of the work of practitioners like you?

Jennifer: (Sigh.) The thing that I would really like is for mothers to claim their right to mother. To claim their competency. I had to do that when my firstborn was five and nearly died. No one else had the right to make the choices that I had the right to make, except his father of course. We've lost that in our culture: women no longer feel that they have the right to mother their children, the right to make those decisions.

When I think now of all the children being taken from their parents, parents who are educated, informed, and who have a spiritual relationship with that child as well. Those pieces come together when that parent makes a decision. Parents don't make the same decision for both of their children in the same circumstance, because they know each individual child. But the medical system wouldn't make those distinctions, or allow for those different decisions. To my mind, we have usurped the humanity that goes into the decision making process. We've laid the parent bare, as if they mean nothing.

I think about my firstborn son in the hospital and the treatment choices I made at that time—nutrition, herbs, homeopathy, acupuncture, bodywork—and I realize that in the world as it is today, they would have taken my child from me. Today, he is a healthy adult, living a full life. (Tears up.) And when we are successful as parents, no one writes about that. You don't read, "Parent made wise medical decision, saved health of child."

Hilary: Jennifer, how can a mother find you, and what do you offer?

Jennifer: My email contact is on my blog, holisticibclc.blogspot.com. I offer a series of webinars to parents about gut healing—"Heal the Mother, Heal the Baby" and another series on "Raising Children Holistically." I see mothers in person or on Skype. And I give a lot of ongoing support to my clients through my private Facebook groups. I also have a series of webinars for professionals on gut healing, airway, holistic lactation, and epigenetics.

Hilary: What would you like to say now to the reader of this book?

Jennifer: Hmmm. I guess would like to say. . . that we have the right to our emotions, to our grief and our joy, and everything in-between.

SHERYL GRUNDE, MOM-BABY YOGA

Doula, licensed massage therapist, yoga instructor,

www.honoringthemother.com

I am Sheryl Grunde, doula, licensed massage therapist and yoga instructor. I have been teaching yoga classes for pregnant women and new moms for the last 13 years in Ashland Oregon. I have two children of my own, 12 and 10 years old.

The postpartum yoga classes that I teach are unique in that they are designed to encourage moms to exercise and socialize while simultaneously playing and interacting with babies as young as six weeks old. We use colorful scarves to captivate the babies' attention and we use sounds to keep them connected to mom and interested in what is going on around them. The babies are lifted and danced with, sung to and massaged. The new moms learn gentle stretches to care for tight shoulders and hips, exercises for strengthening pelvic floor and core muscles, and movements that build strength and feel great. They learn to take care of themselves while continuing to engage with their baby.

New moms are often so focused on their baby's needs that they neglect their own. It is difficult to find time to exercise, but incredibly beneficial for a new mother to connect with her body. So many of the moms remark during their first class that they haven't moved or stretched like that in weeks, and that it feels incredible.

Exercise is one of the simplest, most natural ways to boost your mood. The brain releases endorphins and other chemicals that make us feel better when the heart rate goes up. Moms in my classes frequently remark that stretching and exercising at home has become less daunting now that they have been to class. They have been using the sounds, scarves, and movements at home, too, making time to play with their babies and at the same time, take care of their bodies.

One of my favorite things is to be at the local park with my own kids and run into three or four moms from postpartum yoga classes past, still getting together. I often hear that Baby Yoga classes were the place that the playgroup or moms group or women's circle originated.

Women meet at prenatal yoga when they are pregnant and experiencing similar transitions in life. They continue on into postpartum classes together, where they share advice on baby wearing, books on getting baby to sleep, and delight as they watch the little ones learn and grow together. They make plans to meet at "Babies in the Library" or down at the park, or they walk to the co-op together after class for a smoothie.

New moms need to be around other new moms. We are social creatures, and we need sympathy, a listening ear, and sometimes advice from other women. This emotional support is necessary, and I am grateful to see that the classes I offer facilitate these connections and friendships.

Sheryl's message for the readers of this book:

As a yoga practitioner for nearly twenty years, I would say that yoga has been the single most helpful thing for me—in keeping my calm, caring for my body, and clearing my head. It is true that raising children, caring for a marriage, maintaining a business and being part of a large community can be overwhelmingly complicated at times. I couldn't do it without my yoga practice. It just feels good. Even on the harder days, two minutes of reaching and breathing and twisting and bending after I get out of bed makes my day better. It may help you, too.

AMANDA HOCHMAN, NATUROPATHIC DOCTOR AND MIDWIFE, PROVIDING CARE FROM PRE-CRADLE TO END OF LIFE

Tongue Tie Release Expert

www.all-paths.com

Amanda Hochman is a Naturopathic Doctor and homebirth midwife. Her mission is to accompany her clients on their life journey, pre-cradle to grave. In some cases, Dr. Hochman is the primary caregiver for three generations of the same family. Dr. Hochman is also the recommended go-to person in town for tongue-tie and lip-tie releases.

Hilary: Babies up and down the Rogue Valley are referred to you for tongue- and lip-tie releases. Can you tell me about that?

Amanda: Yes, I often see ties that weren't properly done the first time that I have to correct, and that can be challenging. I prefer if it is only done once, naturally.

It's interesting. . . in a small town such as this one, I can make observations about tongue-tie that are intriguing. For instance, I see more babies from certain doctor's offices, so I know that these doctors are not doing the procedure properly. But I wonder about the other doctors. Are they doing the procedure well, or are they not diagnosing the ties so their mothers are weaning or struggling?

One doctor in town has an excellent approach to nutrition. She works with an in-office nutritionist who personalizes and adjusts a mother's diet for each stage of pregnancy. She has also created a prenatal vitamin that contains folate instead of folic acid, and methyl-B12 instead of cyano-B12. I sometimes wonder if the reason I see no babies from her office is because her nutritional programs and vitamins actually prevent tongue-tie.

Hilary: It would be a great line of research.

Amanda: Yes, it would. Another thing: Lately, I see a lot of baby boys with tongue-tie who also have been diagnosed with phimosis, that is, a tight foreskin over the head of the penis, that will potentially also need to be released. When you see both together, a lot, you have to wonder.

Hilary: Are you able to do follow-up on these babies, to see if the procedure holds?

Amanda: Usually the baby returns for a second visit. If not, the lactation consultant calls and gives me an update. I frequently hear, "The baby gained a pound in a week," where before, they were "failure to thrive". So, yes, I have follow-up, initially.

However, most babies who are referred for a release remain with their primary caregiver, so I don't have a chance to see their long-term results. And that's too bad, I'd like to see their oral development in a few years time.

Hilary: What made you decide to specialize in tongue-tie release?

Amanda: It's because this procedure—it is such a quick thing, a little thing—and it makes a huge difference on many areas of a child's life.

For instance, I often see both tongue and upper-lip ties, and when you release lip-ties you reduce dental carries. I've seen a lot of kids with early tooth decay from nighttime nursing, because the milk collects in the pocket by the tie. So I'm saving a breastfeeding relationship, but I'm also preventing dental carries, and improving many other health areas as well.

Hilary: This is a book about breastfeeding grief. Do you see mothers struggling with emotions around breastfeeding difficulties in your practice?

Amanda: I do see breastfeeding grief in my practice. I see lots of mothers who are struggling to trust that their body is making enough milk. I also see mothers who need help with positioning, finding a position that works for them. But one mother in particular comes to mind for your book.

We tend to think that nursing improves bonding between a mother and her baby. But this mother actually felt that she could not bond with her babies until she stopped nursing and went to a bottle. She felt depressed while breastfeeding. She felt that she couldn't give of herself physically and at the same time be present emotionally for her kids. When she switched to the bottle, her depression resolved, and her interactions with her other children that were challenging became easier.

I gave her some counseling. I let her know that it was okay to make that choice, and that her happiness was the main point.

I think that her experience is true of a lot of mothers, especially those who have assault or abuse histories. When we have these events in our past, when we were forced to surrender control of our body, we want to be able to say in our present life, "My body is my own and I don't have to give it up to you, even for breastfeeding."

Hilary: Yet, it is difficult to bottle-feed by choice today. Our society doesn't really leave room for that.

Amanda: Especially in this town. Here, Moms who need to bottle-feed feel ashamed and embarrassed. They become isolated and might not even leave the house—and that's a big problem.

For me, it's the happiness of the whole family that is my focus, and not the details, not whether breast or bottle. If bottle-feeding is what this mom needed to cope and to be the best mom that she could be, that's what is important. And she felt really relieved to have somebody say that.

Hilary: What would you like to say to the reader?

Amanda: I would say, remember that no matter what, you come first. Because if we are not happy as moms, or within our self, nobody in our house is going to be happy.

I see many mothers who are forty, sixty, seventy years old, still putting others first—and they are looking back, wondering where their life has gone.

I think the biggest thing we can reclaim is to have that deep conversation between our own self and whatever is divine in our world. To really understand what it is that we need to be well.

So I would say, have this conversation. Society's voice is in one ear and out the other most of the time, but having this conversation will allow you to gain a lot throughout your life experience.

Stephanie Pearson,
Researcher, Educator, Essential Oils for Mothers and Babies and Children

http://www.dailynectaressentials.com

Hilary: Hi Stephanie, tell us about yourself. What hats do you wear?

Stephanie: I'm a wellness consultant, a writer, a functional nutritionist, an herbalist, and a wife and mother. But those things are really more about what I do rather than who I am. At heart, I am a researcher and an educator. I love that I have the opportunity to study what I'm passionate about (wellness) and to work with my favorite people (new moms, babies, and children).

My educational path has been 100% navigated by a desire to study subjects that I am most interested in with teachers who inspire me. My degree is in English Literature and Environmental Studies. Postgraduate work includes clinical-level science and health coursework, as well as twenty-five years of botanical medicine study, also outside the classroom and cross-culturally, enriched by field studies in Native American, Western Eclectic, and Latin American herbalism.

Hilary: What motivated you to become a practitioner in essential oils and to focus on the mother and baby?

Stephanie: I struggled so much as a new mother and then again when coping with a chronically sick toddler. This was when my children were very young and before we moved back to Portland to be closer to my parents. Most of our friends were in graduate school and my husband was working 50 hours a week. I had severe sleep issues in postpartum that dramatically decreased my quality of life. It took over a year to regain my stamina. I learned so much about using nutrition and herbs to improve my own health that I went back to school so that I could fill this need for someone else, to make sure that no woman had to endure a difficult postpartum without support or needlessly.

Hilary: How do you help mothers who are going through breastfeeding grief?

Stephanie: One of the best gifts that we can give to someone who is struggling is our undivided attention and to listen without judgment. Essential oils (EO) can help dramatically as well, and are so easy to use. When used aromatically, essential oils go straight to the limbic system where they have the potential to balance neurotransmitters, affect endocrine organs, and even help to release stored trauma from the amygdala. Mothers who are struggling with any aspect of breastfeeding, or who are struggling with the emotional part of these challenges, or who are highly fatigued, depressed or emotional, unable to breastfeed for whatever reason, can feel supported and balanced with EO.

Hilary: And finally, what would you like to say to the reader of this book.

Stephanie: The three best ways that I've found to get through a difficult time are to spend time walking in nature, to write down everything for which you are grateful, and to use essential oils to support yourself in getting through the difficult moments. Herbs are our allies and will be there for you whenever you need some help.

HILARY JACOBSON,
HOLISTIC BREASTFEEDING CONSULTANT
CLINICAL HYPNOTHERAPIST, CERTIFIED MEDICAL SPECIALIST

healingbreastfeedinggrief.com, mother-food.com

Ever since I struggled through breastfeeding grief, thirty years ago, I have felt motivated to help mothers heal from their breastfeeding traumas.

It is heartbreaking to look forward to motherhood, to do your very best to be prepared, and then to have the rug pulled out from under you— precisely at the moment you want nothing more than to be a solid, positive presence for your baby.

Hypnotherapy enables mothers to quickly let go of the stress of negative feelings and thoughts and to build positive, relaxed emotional states that build confidence and connection, and that empower mothers to embark on their healing journeys.

On my website healingbreastfeedinggrief.com, you can contact me to book an appointment. Also, check out my listing of hypnotherapists who have training and experience to work with mothers after childbirth. Most hypnotherapists today work per Skype as well as in person, so you don't have to leave your home to receive this support. The website also features articles about subjects discussed in this book, updates on new publications, new interviews, videos and webinars, and a list of online support groups and specialized therapies for breastfeeding problems.

Please join my Facebook group Healing Breastfeeding Grief to meet with other mothers and share stories and healing experiences.

Testimonials from Clients

J.H., a first-time mother.

"Working with Hilary on milk supply and also hypnotherapy around issues of increasing milk, traumatic birth and adjusting to motherhood has been a major part of my healing process. Hilary is kind and gentle, and she truly cares for the wellbeing of others. She deeply understands these issues and the range of the emotions that go along with them. I was not so sure about doing hypnotherapy by phone but it actually worked out great to do it in a familiar space (home) by phone. She helped me come up with follow-up work to do on my own which felt very manageable for a new mother (while falling asleep and in the shower!).

"My brain and heart healed tremendously through this work. I feel a lot stronger now and am loving being a mom to my baby girl. It was a huge adjustment, the challenging birth, and a lot to sort through in my mind, and in the end, all of it was worth it. I have never known love to be so deep as with a child. It's a new miracle every day. I am grateful to Hilary for her easy, caring way and all of the knowledge that she has acquired and is willing to share on these topics. I highly recommend her hypnotherapy to anyone who has gone through a traumatic birth and/or dealing with milk issues."

C.H., a mother, after the birth of her second child.

"Hilary enabled me to regain a part of myself I thought was gone, something I had given up on altogether. I have since been able to encounter old, pervasive problems with a whole new understanding, unusual patience and success."

M.G. sister of a mother of three.

"My sister is a client of yours. With her permission and encouragement, I am writing to let you know that I have noticed a phenomenal difference in her over the past several months. She is more and more becoming the woman I have always known was there under the veil of past trauma and severe self-criticism. I notice it in small things she says; ways she speaks about life, about herself, about our parents. In a nutshell, she feels more clear and self-confident—and like she knows she is deserving of that. This is the first time in my life that I have witnessed her this way. Thank you thank you thank you for the gift you have given my sister."

M. M., mother of two beautiful boys.

"Hilary is a gifted woman. I would recommend her to anyone. I was skeptical at first about hypnotherapy, but during (what I thought was) a casual conversation, I was already dropping emotional baggage like anvils, as problems I had been struggling with seemed to just slip away. That was 5 months ago and I can't thank you enough Hilary!"

THREE MOTHERS SHARE THEIR STORIES
BEKKI H.

Before my first child was born, I didn't think about breastfeeding very much. I watched my own mother breastfeed my six younger siblings. It was just a normal act of mothering, like changing diapers and kissing boo-boos. Because breastfeeding is such a natural thing to do, I didn't even bother taking any breastfeeding classes. I assumed that my primal instinct to feed my child would kick in, and that my body would just do what it was made to do.

After an exceptionally long labor and subsequent cesarean section, I knew that there could be a delay in my milk. But my daughter lost weight at an alarming rate, and the lactation consultant recommended supplementing. I supplemented with a tube to avoid bottles for the first couple of weeks, held her skin-to-skin, nursed around the clock, and pumped whenever possible. Still, my milk never came in, and my daughter continued to lose weight. The more I increased the amount of her supplement, the more I felt like a failure as a mother.

I received a great deal of support from my family and local community. Lactation consultants, doulas, La Leche League Leaders—they all rallied around me to help me feed my baby, and they were all left scratching their heads, with no idea as to what was wrong.

After a few weeks, I was diagnosed with mammary hypoplasia. I learned that my breasts lack sufficient mammary tissue to produce enough milk to sustain a baby. I followed a strict lactogenic diet and consumed copious amounts of galactagogues to increase the little bit that I did produce. But the regretful feeling of not being enough always hung over me like a dark cloud.

My doula connected me with a colleague of hers who had a surplus of pumped breastmilk in her freezer. This woman shared her stash, so that I could supplement with human milk, rather than commercial formula. From there, I connected with a milksharing network, where I found other donors who generously shared their milk with me, so that my baby would not go without. Their love and kindness was the fuel that got me through many difficult days.

When my daughter was four months old, I became overwhelmed with grief over not producing enough. My routine of nursing, supplementing and pumping became unbearably strenuous, and I was ready to throw in the towel and quit all together. I called and cried to my mother, who encouraged me not to give up. She recommended that I stop pressuring myself to make every drop of milk possible, and instead just enjoy the milk that I did make. She reassured me that it didn't have to be all or nothing.

Shifting my focus from quantity to quality made a tremendous difference. We continued to breastfeed, without the stress and guilt of low production. But when my baby rejected the breast at eight months old and our breastfeeding relationship ended too soon, the dark feelings resurfaced. I was left emotionally devastated.

With my second child, I convinced myself that things would be better. Rather than focusing on what I knew I could achieve and working with that, I put all of my hopes in a dream that I logically knew was out of my reach—a full milk supply, and breastfeeding without supplement. This failure to hold realistic expectations brought on even worse grief than the first time around, as I watched yet another one of my babies rapidly lose weight on my supply. I employed the same arsenal of milk boosting tools— skin-to-skin, frequent nursing, frequent pumping, herbs, lactogenic foods— worked myself in to the ground until I became exhausted. At four months, my son began rejecting the breast, and refused to nurse. I became depressed. I felt like I was not a good enough mother, because I couldn't provide my babies with one of their most basic needs—nourishment.

My son was blessed with donor milk just as his sister had been. During my pregnancy with him, I connected with a local donor who produced enough excess in a day to feed more than two babies. She filled my freezer with her milk before he was even born. Shortly after his arrival, she moved all the way across the country, but she wanted to continue to provide milk for him. She shipped milk thousands of miles on a regular basis. We both had some experience with shipping milk, but over the months we perfected our technique. Word traveled on the Internet of our breastmilk shipping endeavors, and several other families contacted us, looking to learn how to do this for themselves.

To save time, we created a blog with instructions on how to safely freeze, pack and ship breastmilk. Our following grew, and we soon became a support group for milksharing families, guiding them on everything from safe milksharing practices to shipping to etiquette. In some rare cases, we personally assisted the families of extremely medically frail babies, making matches and finding milk for these babies, because their parents were too busy caring for them in the hospital.

One day, one of these mothers told me, "Thank you. My baby would have died without breastmilk. You saved my baby's life."

That was when I realized that all of the heartbreak and devastation I had suffered had eventually resulted in something beautiful. Having been through this low milk supply journey, I learned valuable skills that could be used to help other people.

Supporting milksharing families has done so much to heal the gaping wounds that I once carried. Taking all of that negative energy and using it for something good has brought much more fulfillment to my life than merely having a full milk supply and feeding my own babies. Even though my breasts lack the ability to feed one baby, I've learned that my heart is capable of helping to feed hundreds. In my own small way.

And in learning how to manage my own low milk supply, I have also educated myself on how to help other women who struggle with feeding their own babies. Helping low milk supply moms became another passion of mine, so I trained to become a Certified Lactation Counselor. I work on a volunteer basis with local moms who struggle to produce milk. If I can't help them achieve the full milk supply that every mother desires, I educate them on how to make the most of what they do produce, and help them get started in milksharing, so that they can supplement with human milk if they desire.

By the time my third child was born, my expectations were much more realistic. I had made peace with my low milk supply and was determined to work with my challenges, not against them.

I brought donor milk to the hospital when I gave birth, so that, from the moment my youngest daughter needed supplementing, she had breastmilk. This took an enormous amount of pressure off of me, as I didn't have to feel concerned with what she was being fed. My baby was eating and growing; that was what was important.

Though we used bottles early on, we mastered the SNS so that she could supplement at the breast. We both found the SNS difficult and stressful to use in the beginning, as many mothers and babies do. With my first two babies, I gave up on the SNS pretty quickly. But with my third, I decided to start out using it part time. I decided to only use it when I felt comfortable, and it didn't cause any anxiety. If a feeding with the SNS felt at all daunting, I would set it aside to try again later, and just supplement with a bottle. After a few weeks of practicing without pressure, we both became quite proficient. Soon, we gave up bottles all together.

Now I have the breastfeeding relationship that I have always dreamed of. I may not make much milk, but thanks to donor milk and the SNS, my little girl doesn't know the difference. And while my first two babies refused the breast at a young age, my littlest one is now a toddler, still nursing, with no end in sight.

Learning how to cope with my breastfeeding grief was a long journey. There were some very dark days, and feelings of inadequacy. Through these experiences, and with patience, acceptance, and by turning pain into a vehicle to help others, I now can't imagine my life without knowing these struggles. They have defined a big part of who I am as a mother, and not in a bad way. I no longer look at myself as the sad, broken mother who could not produce. Rather, I see a strength that I didn't know I possessed. I just had to do a little digging to find it.

ARIELLE

My journey into motherhood started with an epic love story and a comfortable, symptom free pregnancy. At 37 years old, still technically obese despite two years of diet and exercise along with a 90-pound weight loss, I was thrilled and surprised by conceiving easily. During pregnancy I became acquainted with the intense love and worry that comes with motherhood. I had the pleasure of having a baby that sat right occiput from 35 weeks on and a placenta placed so perfectly that I never got a single uncomfortable kick to a lung or rib, so I could not feel the baby moving unless he did a full roll back and forth. The lack of sensing movement when I was being advised to do daily fetal movement counts gave me tremendous anxiety for several weeks prior to birth. This was the beginning of my understanding the bond between mother and child, this time where you must tune in and listen quietly for instinct to lead you into assurance that all is well, or the realization that there is truly something wrong,.

There was intense celebration and excitement throughout the pregnancy, as I was just married to my husband David, my best friend, and we were moving to a new state to start our journey as a family. I focused on a healthy diet and exercise, had an excellent prenatal healthcare experience, a supportive partner, quality prenatal vitamins, followed the Schuessler cell salt protocol for pregnancy and lactation, you name it, I was prepared to do everything to the best of my ability. We named our son Alfred and started talking to him and playing relaxing classical music for him as soon as his little ears had formed. He had a few tunes that he particularly loved so I hummed them to him regularly.

David and I got all the support structures we thought we'd need in place, knowing it would greatly improve my birth experience and transition to motherhood. We had a wonderful doula that was competent in all birthing techniques from acupressure and yoga to homeopathy and aromatherapy. We had a birth plan including alternatives so that we were mentally prepared for any decisions we might need to make should things go awry. David faithfully attended every class offered by our birthing hospital from infant massage and CPR to yoga for delivery and breastfeeding.

We were thrilled with their hands off approach to labor and delivery. They practice kangaroo care, delayed cord clamping, and had a great lactation support staff in place that does not offer formula. My Obstetrician respected all of my birth plan decisions. I had my breast pump, custom fit flanges and nursing pillow packed into my hospital bag so I was ready to go. I had it all covered down to having immediate family at home for the first few weeks to help support us. My sister had told my husband exactly how to plan a nursing vacation for me so that all I would need to do was feed the baby and rest.

On a certain conscious level I was ready for and expecting an easy natural birth just like my mother had experienced. We enjoyed many lengthy discussions about birthing practices and what to expect after birthing a child, but problems nursing did not come up in conversation as she had an easy time of it. Her best advice was to put a waterproof cover on our mattress for when the water would break because it was her experience that it always happens when you are sleeping. Low and behold that is exactly what happened, on Mother's Day evening during a full moon. I was excited to wake up at 2am to my water slowly leaking. Our doula had instructed us to stay home as long as possible through the contractions. I slept until 5am, woke up my husband and told him we'd be having the baby soon, then told him to go back to sleep and to take a long hot shower as we were not going to rush.

I went downstairs and fed myself a huge breakfast of leftover Mother's Day foods in preparation for the birthing experience. I was at 38 weeks and had an Obstetric checkup scheduled that morning at 10am. I called when they opened and was told to bring my hospital bag as I would be admitted if it was amniotic fluid. After that phone call I noticed a pair of sparrows trapped in our newly constructed screened-in porch so I rushed out with a light towel in hand ready to catch them gently and release them outside the porch. I quickly realized they had slipped in under the doors as the door strips were not yet installed. I managed to lead the male bird out the door and was in the process of doing the same for the mother sparrow when my husband came upon the scene. It was a comical moment for us when he saw me running around the porch chasing birds while waiting to go into labor. I managed to get the mama bird gently into the towel and released her outside, she met her mate at their nest and I wished her well.

In all of this time I did not have any contractions but I expected them to come at any moment. They never came. My husband loaded the car and we went to our appointment to confirm that the water had broken. Indeed, I had a premature rupture of membrane but at 38 weeks, so we checked into the hospital for labor and delivery.

My birth did not go as planned but the birth itself was a wonderful experience. We had an amazing doula that helped my husband and me maximize our chances for a natural birth. There was a walking fetal monitor so I had free reign to walk about the hospital in an effort to stimulate contractions. We tried every single tool in the arsenal, but 24 hours later there was still not a single contraction. We decided to be induced, and Pitocin gave me such strong contractions that an epidural was an easy choice. My Obstetrician let me and my husband be in full control of our birthing choices. That was a great feeling. We spent the majority of my labor watching the Saturday morning cartoons of our childhoods and eating our favorite cooked sushi rolls. We had great music and aromatherapy going. Because of this freedom to create our own experience, even with the changes to our birth plan I felt that it was *my* birth.

As humans, we respond to smell, color and imagery with all the cells of our body. I know this experience as an artist, too. Imagery touches me to the core. Once I was fully dilated, I asked for the rose oil out of the aromatherapy kit I had packed, and inhaling its scent I visualized a vivid red rose blooming, gently unfolding to the beautiful yellow center at its heart. In that heart was my child. Much to the surprise and delight of our birthing team our son Alfie came into the world with only ten full strength pushes.

Witnessing this beautiful miracle was the most incredible moment of my life. The nurses had set up a mirror so I could watch his progress toward crowning and his actual birth. Alfie, created within, here at last and face to face. He was peaceful on my chest as David and I soaked him in.

He latched and nursed immediately with that sleepy, early term baby kind of nursing at first. After a while David cut the cord and the nurses took Alfie to a table about four feet away to do the APGAR scoring—and he began to wail. I started to hum his favorite tune and he turned his head in my direction and stopped crying immediately. The Labor and Delivery nurse took one look at me and said, "Well this one definitely knows who his mama is." That line has always stuck with me. I realized our bond was inseparable even as our bodies had become separate.

The birth was an early morning one so we could enjoy three days at the hospital for recovery. We had a team of wonderful caregivers. Each nurse gave me her favorite swaddling, diapering and burping methods. The lactation consultants were amazing. They saw that breastfeeding was important to me, and that I was prepared to work. Alfie was a sleepy early term baby with a week latch at first so I had to wake him often to nurse. I was told to pump ten times a day and to nurse every 2 hours at minimum. They showed me how to collect colostrum with a syringe and, when he was not latching well, to give it to him as he suckled on my finger. At one point the lactation consultants told me he needed help latching as I had very small 16mm nipples that would not stay erect and he was having a hard time positioning to latch. We used Thera shells and nipple shields that were correctly fit and his latch improved immensely.

With a working nursing relationship in place we were sent home. At our first pediatric visit seven days post-partum, Alfie had not put on enough weight, so we were told to come back for a weigh-in at ten days post-partum. At our ten day appointment we were told that Alfie wasn't putting on weight adequately and we were advised to supplement along with nursing, and to follow up quickly with an IBCLC. Fortunately, our pediatrician's office has several doctors and they are all IBCLC's. I soon found out that not many had experience with low supply, and I saw several before I found the right one. When I found her, it was a godsend.

She evaluated Alfie's latch and determined he was transferring well despite a very mild tongue-tie and upper lip-tie. She also asked me to do labs to determine the cause of my suppressed lactation. She showed me how using a larger nipple shield would widen and deepen his latch as it got stronger, and how to easily wean off the nipple shield. We did weighed feeds and saw that Alfie was transferring two ounces each session. I was really happy to find out that he was transferring more than my maximum output from pumping. A nurse in her office had experienced low supply and the grief it causes, so my doctor had me sit down and talk with her, as someone who could relate to my experience. I found that connection cathartic, and also sought out an amazing Low Milk Supply group on Facebook so that I had other mothers with my experience to speak with. The group had a wealth of information in its files regarding my reasons for suppressed lactation.

My sister Vivienne was a wonderful cheerleader for me as I struggled to learn and incorporate all these techniques in the midst of the sleep deprived hormonal storm that is early post-partum. Vivienne reached out to my local La Leche League and got the contact information for a wonderful woman who came to my house and further helped me. This woman also sent me in-depth articles on nipple shields and how to wean off of them when the baby is ready. The techniques worked like a charm. All of this extra work on top of nursing, supplementing and pumping around the clock, actually made me feel relieved, because we were using everything correctly.

At 5 weeks Alfie was off the nipple shields and was nursing contently. Sometimes he wanted a bottle supplement after nursing and other times he fell asleep full and content. Our next visit to our pediatrician was wonderful, as he had been gaining weight beautifully since we started supplementing at ten days old. Now that he was weaned from nipple shields an SNS was suggested, but I have an allergy to adhesives so I chose to bottle supplement.

When my IBCLC who is also Alfie's pediatrician saw how upset I was with having low supply, she helped me begin reframing my experience. She said very compassionately: "Your baby will get all the benefits and immunity of your milk from you, and he will get all the calories he needs from formula." That began my gratitude toward formula and having a healthy, hungry baby. I seriously love that woman. She was a godsend to me and taught me how to persevere happily.

Alfie and I got into a good routine of nursing, pumping and sleeping from five weeks on. David was an incredible partner through all of this. He stood by me and supported me both emotionally and physically with tons of hands-on help. He kept a stock of water, fruits and nuts by my big comfy nursing chair in the living room as well as on my night table upstairs. We both did a lot of baby wearing with skin-to-skin and focused on all of the recommended techniques to recreate the feeling of the womb for our little Alfie to feel loved and content. We had a happy easy baby and were in the swing of things, or so I thought.

Looking back, I was like that frantic mama sparrow trapped in my porch the morning of Alfie's birth. There was a primal scream just under the surface that I was keeping at bay. MY BABY IS STARVING. It was not in words, but in every cell of my body there was stress. It manifested in feelings of inadequacy and anxiety, as well as negative self-image. My body was betraying me in the worst way imaginable. It was starving my baby. If we did not have formula he would not survive. *I was not enough for him.* I did all that work to lose 90 pounds before getting married and I put it all back on during pregnancy. I was a failure. I could not relax at all. I was not enjoying motherhood and my child the way I wanted to.

I became angry—and I am very glad I became angry because I started to let that primal scream course through my body and it started to find its way out. First it was hypervigilence with tracking Alfie's food intake and then it was research into the causes and treatments for my suppressed lactation. Why was I incapable of producing more than half of my son's milk? I discovered I had low prolactin and insulin resistance, both of which were interfering with the delicate hormone balances required for lactation. I began correcting my diet by reducing carbohydrates and by focusing on quality ingredients. I also started exercising daily, just simple walks in the sunshine with Alfie in my carrier or stroller.

I started meditating on these walks, drawing on techniques for breathing and visualizing I had learned in my college years. I prayed to find peace, as well, and it started to find me as I let out that frantic mama scream I was holding back in small doses each time I walked. I breathed in a healing golden light from well above my head and let it fill my body as the warm sunshine caressed my skin. I let the light flow down and out of the soles of my feet, pushing out the negativity as it coursed through every cell. I let it out, sending it deep into the ground where it could rest peacefully as it was done. My legs became firmly planted roots and I began to feel strong. Now I began to enjoy every moment with Alfie. I would spend hours watching him nap on my chest. I cherished every single moment.

At three months I stopped pumping and started meditating as I nursed. I would visualize that soft rosy pink color of love emanating from my heart and wrapping around my son. The fact that I supplemented with a bottle of formula stopped bothering me because I just knew that our connection was stronger than what filled his belly. I actually started to enjoy bottle feeding and felt grateful that I could fill his food need and watch him sleep peacefully on a full belly. I learned a lot in the first three months, but I learned a lot more once I became fully present. I could easily tend to his needs, read his body language and cues because I was at peace. This experience set me up for my kind of mothering. Things will not be perfect, but I will be there doing my best and I will stay present, in the moment, for my family.

We continued on through the typical nursing strikes and the distractions of a curious baby becoming ever more aware of his surroundings and had a successful nursing relationship for fifteen months. I loved bedsharing and night nursing. As he got a few months older and I introduced solids I did not need to supplement at night, and we slept so peacefully in a relaxed lazy night nursing rhythm. I even froze milk for after he weaned so I could supplement with my own milk. Today, Alfie is almost two years old and we still nurse on occasion. He likes falling asleep with skin-to-skin, and will even stop playing periodically through the day to snuggle and rub my belly. It's just so sweet, and reassuring to know that my body and my presence helps him find his center, helps him ground and feel secure.

All of the work and struggle was worth it, and I would not change this experience. It taught me about my emotional self and helped me focus on processing emotions in a healthy way. I learned about insulin resistance and have lost those ninety pounds. I now have the knowledge to prevent diabetes and heart disease, which progress from insulin resistance. I would have never known about this if I didn't have a low milk supply.

I have always been the type of person who would find the good in a situation but this was the deepest experience of self-growth I have had to date. It could not have happened at a better time. I am a stronger person, and have a genuine loving presence to offer my son. I am confident that I am enough.

CANDY

I come from a long line of breastfeeding women, going back to my great grandmother and including my mother, my many aunts and my sisters. They were all breastfed and able to breastfeed, and I was breastfed until I was two and a half years old. Was it too much to assume that I would be able to breastfeed too, in spite of my oddly shaped breasts?

I shared my concerns with my Ob-Gyn when my breasts didn't grow or change during pregnancy, but she was very busy and didn't respond to my question. I also took a class in breastfeeding. None of the problems I would have were covered in that class, and not one of the medical professionals who observed my oddly shaped breasts during pregnancy offered an opinion or mentioned a possible impact on my ability to nurse.

Finally, the big day came. My water broke. But I didn't have contractions. My doctor said I should check in to hospital, just to be safe. I had a birth plan, printed in triplicate, and I handed it out to the attending nurses. My plan stated that no drugs were to be used.

Soon, a nurse spoke vaguely about "helping along the contractions." Suddenly, I was subjected to an IV and given a small amount of "stimulant" as they told me. It was Pitocin.

From then on, my labor was out of my hands. I was pressured, laughed at for my birth plan, never told to relax my body, made to lay down on my back, and the Pitocin was increased from my agreed level of 2 drops up to what I would later discover was 27.

I was furious, anxious and concerned about the effect of the medication on my baby. I was in a state of constant contraction. It was so bad that I agreed to an epidural, just so I could relax.

Finally, I was coached to push and I received my beautiful son into my arms. He latched right away, and I believed we were off to a good start.

But then came the lethargy—my son slept and slept. No wonder, after all the medications. The nurse instructed me to breastfeed once every three to four hours. I had to wake him for every feed and keep a feeding log that they checked off and Okayed.

I nursed once every four hours, under the eyes of the nurses, while my son mostly slept at the breast and I didn't notice any real swallowing!

This hospital is certified "Baby Friendly." But I believe they use that to attract clients. By day three, he had lost 9% of his birth weight, my milk hadn't come in, and a nurse pressured me to supplement with formula before I left the hospital.

Every day thereafter, my son had to go back to the hospital for a blood test. The trip exhausted him, and he was becoming jaundiced. At night I rocked him as he cried in hunger. I still did not know that I should nurse him when he prompted, and not according to when the hospital schedule permitted.

A week after he was born, my nipples were chafed, scabbed and bloody. Nursing made me cry from pain. I began to research problems like tongue-tie, and I suspected this was an issue for my son. But his pediatrician insisted he wasn't tongue-tied. He said my son's latch "just wasn't right" and that I needed to make a better breast-sandwich or whatever. Well, my son's tongue wouldn't move beyond his gums, and today, at nearly three years old, his tongue can't stick out without being cleft in the middle from the tightness of his frenulum.

The lactation consultants at the hospital told me I needed to supplement while I used a breast pump to increase my supply. They recommended that I use More Milk Plus tincture—the worst thing I had ever tasted but it did prove to be effective.

Breastfeeding my baby completely defined motherhood for me then. With a big pump, the tincture, and, finally, some good advice to breastfeed more often, I felt that I could make it work. I still didn't know about hypoplasia or insufficient glandular tissue.

I pumped 14 times a day, nursed 10 times a day, and supplemented with formula that I injected with a syringe into the side of my son's mouth. I had no uninterrupted sleep for weeks. My measured pumped milk was 16 ounces a day at my peak. I measured my output obsessively. Milliliters less than expected would send me crashing into hysteria.

I felt like the most pathetic person—a worthless fraud of a mother. Even my husband was afraid to discuss anything with me since I was so easily set off. Then began my endless research: I used breast compression during pumping and nursing, massage, hot showers, hot rice packs, every tincture, tea and food I heard about. I tried to relax...but that never happened, I was so desperate.

Then I began to learn about breast hypoplasia and it broke me again. I felt deformed, insufficient, worthless, pathetic, like I had no business being a mother. My family took pity on me and told me it was okay to give up. Then my mother suggested La Leche League. I attended, but they couldn't tell me more than I was already trying. They said they had never encountered someone with problems like mine before. I felt so alone.

That changed when I discovered the book "A Breastfeeding Mother's Guide to Making More Milk." I was not alone! Many mothers had problems like mine. And when I read that mothers went on to have a full supply with later babies, I had hope again.

During this whole time I also stressed over formula and their use of cheap, inferior ingredients. We had purchased one type that was designed to alleviate gas and were in horror as the first three and hence major ingredients were low quality sugars. It was returned.

I then searched for and actually found a breastmilk donor who had exactly the amount of extra milk per day that I lacked. And, thankfully, she would become an ongoing donor. I bought a box of 400 milk bags for her. I traveled 100 mile round trips 3 times every 2 months. I brought gifts of quality food and garden raised veggies to my donor mom. My gratitude was endless.

For eight months, until just after my son turned one, I could feed my son at my breasts using an SNS, using the donated milk. At that point, I stopped supplementing. Since he was eating plenty and drinking other fluids, I was able to breastfeed him on what I could make. I happily celebrated nursing for another thirteen months with only my own supply. Every request to nurse by my son was a triumph, accompanied by pure elation.

When my son was eighteen months old, I was pregnant again. I started to research how to ensure better lactation. I came across Hilary Jacobson's book "Mother Food" and began to compile foods, herbs, begin breast massage, and drink my own blend of teas for different stages of pregnancy. I also made my own tinctures—but they all tasted worse than the first tincture I had bought.

I had a wonderful natural birth at a birth center and felt amazing afterwards. My new son was a nursing pro with no tongue-tie. Lots of colostrum was flowing. I was taking all my supplements, and I felt hopeful that I was going to breastfeed exclusively.

Then came the complications.

I had to take my son to a clinic for a blood draw, and it was done so poorly that the results were compromised. I had been strep B positive and hadn't received antibiotics due to my very rapid labor, so his blood tests were extremely important to the medical community. With inconclusive results, the new pediatrician told us to go to the emergency room. When admitted, they treated us like crazy hippies for going to a birthing center. They drew his blood via IV, and then left in the IV. Then a doctor told us our son would have to be admitted, put on oxygen, given antibiotics, have a spinal tap, and be tested hourly just in case he might be infected. During the next hour, my son was forcibly held down and strapped into an arm sling with a huge IV port that was taped to a splint. He was two days old and totally frightened.

Now, Strep B early onset manifests immediately, and he had no signs of fever, lethargy, etc. My husband and I argued with the doctor. We insisted that we wait for the correct blood test results. The pressure was laid on us to comply with the doctor, but fortunately the pediatrician reported back about the blood test: my son was fine, we could go home.

Tragically, due to this terrifying ordeal, my son slept non-stop during the next two days when my milk came in. My breasts were very full. I had to wake my baby constantly to feed him, but he would just fall asleep on the breast. I was panicking.

On the sixth day of his life, my son was becoming jaundiced. Soon it was clear that he wasn't getting enough milk. I was very upset. Whether it was due to my still insufficient glands or to the medical intervention, I couldn't know for sure. I just knew that the critical days had been wasted.

I was down and devastated again. I had hoped that with hard work and lots of help from natural remedies and great advice I could make it work. Not so.

However, I did have one consolation. I had found a wonderful formula, full of amazing ingredients that are well researched, healthy, and unprocessed. With lots of pumping and using a hospital grade pump, I reached 18 oz at my peak.

Then the phone call came. About two months into my son's life, the donor mom who helped out with my first son wanted to know if I had perchance had another baby. She had just had her second child the same week my son was born and she had the same oversupply. I was so happy, stunned and blessed. My baby would have 100% breastmilk. Not only that, but both my sons would have the same milk donor.

I celebrated by making the trip, getting the milk and supplementing my son! It was wonderful. I had become calm again, accepting of my insufficiency, for now. The milk donations lasted for three months before my donor mom had an unexpected job loss and stopped pumping. We stretched the last batch of milk out for two months, using it as a once-a-week treat, or during illness.

I am looking forward to the next experience with breastfeeding. I have resigned myself to the fact that I have a limited supply due to a flaw in my anatomy, which I may or may not be able to change. I have gone through meltdowns and extreme highs due to supply problems. I have grieved over my bizarre breasts, and my children's deficit of ideal nutrition as young babies. But, I have also realized that because I was so determined, so unwilling to give up when the situation was so bleak, and when the advice was bad, that I did win in the end, and I did breastfeed my sons.

Addendum... Six months later. He is 16 months now. I've finally reached that calm, quiet, joyous, peaceful time in our nursing relationship, where the communication, closeness and comfort is the primary benefit to us both. Yet, most nights, as he stirs and nurses, I do wake up and consciously wait to hear him swallow milk. I'm still thinking in measurements and am still excited to know I am producing anything at all. I mentally count the seconds where he is actively swallowing as a way to boost my confidence and remind myself I really worked hard for this.

I did something very therapeutic this holiday season; I wanted to share it with you because, well, you'll see...

I wanted to give something to all my sisters. I made tiny nativity ornaments from clay that, when I began creating them, were very typical of the traditional nativity scene, kneeling parents, baby in a manger, but they progressed by the third ornament to Mary lying down next to Jesus, and then to Mary nursing and co-sleeping. Joseph is also more relaxed, often reclined and usually touching the baby or Mary, very close and focused.

I am never more in awe of my children and of life than when I hold my soft, warm babies against my body, and I feel that Mary would have been reverent whilst nursing and holding her baby, too.

I painted all the ceramic nativities after I fired them in the kiln and they came out great. My family all enjoyed them and I had to save several for myself of course. Looking at them gives me a joy that is similar to the success of breastfeeding, because both are labor of love and faith, hope and joy.

I would also like to add that through all the supplementation issues and devices, and my highs and lows, my sons preferred to nurse, cuddle and require me for their nourishment as well as for comfort. The fact that this was their preference and desire, and that they continued breastfeeding because they wanted to, reinforced my drive and reassured me that I had done the right thing for all of us.

FOR RESOURCES, UPDATES AND INFORMATION

Join Hilary Jacobson at www.healingbreastfeedinggrief.com or www.mother-food.com for resources, new publications, articles, webinars, interviews and stories.

Find Hilary Jacobson on Facebook at her Mother Food Page and her group Healing Breastfeeding Grief.

ENDNOTES

---

[i]Borra, C., Iacovou, M. and Sevilla, A. "New Evidence on Breastfeeding and Postpartum Depression: The Importance of Understanding Women's Intentions". Maternal and Child Health Journal: 20 Aug 2014

[ii]Gallup Jr., GG et al. Bottle feeding simulates child loss: Postpartum depression and evolutionary medicine. Med Hypotheses (2009), doi: 10.1016/j.mehy.2009.07.016

[iii] http://www.ima.org.il/imaj/ViewArticle.aspx?aId=147

Printed in Great Britain
by Amazon